Foreword

They are called 'refugees', 'asylum seekers', 'queue jumpers', and 'displaced persons', but no matter how they are referred to these are always the names of 'others'. Unless you have lived these names it is hard, if not impossible, to know how difficult your life could be, or how detrimental this state of being could be to your health.

The Health of Refugees: Public Health Perspectives from Crisis to Settlement brings home some of the realities facing refugees around the world, and in particular those who have arrived on our Australian shores. It does so in many, complementary ways; objectively in clear expositions, using epidemiological, clinical and sociological evidence, but also by telling private, heart-wrenching stories of refugees, many of whom have not only endured much suffering to get to Australia, but who continue to face humiliation after they have arrived.

The authors provide clear arguments for how to change the way we are currently doing business, described in one chapter as 'suspending the development of one subgroup by restricting the capacity of its members to participate meaningfully in society'. The book also gives clear directions about the way forward such as developing a 'consistent nationwide network of health services' to cater for immigrants and refugees, 'regardless of entry category'.

This important book should be mandatory reading for policy makers, clinicians, health promoters, lawyers, social workers, teachers, undergraduate students, academics, and local government organisers who work with new arrivals. It forms a critical mass of information in an area that, up until now, has been difficult to access.

The Health of Refugees: Public Health Perspectives from Crisis to Settlement is a timely and valuable contribution to our knowledge of broad public-health issues, as well as the even broader context in which refugees find themselves in contemporary Australia. It reminds us that, despite the predominant fear of refugee movements in wealthy countries such as Australia, it is developing countries such as Pakistan, Iran, and Tanzania that cope with the truly enormous burdens of migration. It also encourages the reader to explore and understand the way in which public opinion is being determined.

Health care for refugees has become a highly contested and divisive issue. Like many key public-health issues it has become 'political' simply because of the divergence of opinion in our community. This book, however, takes an overtly 'Hippocratic' stand in defence of the basic human right to health care.

Written by authors who not only care about the people they are working with, but who also care about the integrity and excellence of their scholarship, this book comes from the heart as well as from the head. Because of this duality the authors' guidance can only produce good results, not only for refugees but also for Australia's health as a whole.

Dr Rob Moodie
Chief Executive Officer
Victorian Health Promotion Foundation (VicHealth)
PO Box 154 Carlton South, Victoria 3053, Australia

The predicament of refugees is a steady reminder that we live in an age of upheaval. What distinguishes our time, aside from the scale and ubiquity of political violence, is that global communities have become interwoven in ways that are orders of magnitude faster, tighter and more compelling than ever before. This raises special issues for the public health response to refugees.

To address these issues, Pascale Allotey and her colleagues have written an important book that takes its place in a small but illustrious lineage that began with Henry Murphy's *Flight and Resettlement*, published by UNESCO in 1955. In that volume, mental health professionals addressed the predicament of displaced peoples in the aftermath of World War II. The emphasis was on the mental health needs of people living in exile. Fifty years on, the refugee situation has been transformed in many ways. The magnitude of the problem has increased, the circumstances of forced displacement and migration have become more diverse, and our knowledge base about migration, health, and trauma has grown. At the same time, the world is being pulled in opposing directions: towards greater integration with lines of communication and exchange transcending borders and, simultaneously, towards erecting barriers, closing doors and denying the legitimacy of claims for asylum.

The creation of the status of refugee by the 1951 convention represented an important moment in the evolution of a more global moral consciousness and commitment that acknowledges our obligation to each other as human beings and inhabitants of one world. The right for asylum is an extension of protection from those living in safety to those exposed to threat—who are distinguished only by accidents of birth.

While earlier generations of immigrants came to countries like Australia, Canada, and the US under circumstances that would make them refugees in today's definition, their predicament differed in some important respects. Many migrated with little hope of maintaining contact or returning to the places they left. They were propelled forward and came to consider their new land their permanent home and invested heavily in the future; the successes of their children gave meaning to their suffering and loss. Today refugees have more possibilities of maintaining contact with their place of origin and, consequently, may feel a sharper sense of exile. To the extent that they and their children face obstacles to permanent settlement and advancement, it may be difficult to move beyond the traumatic rupture of their lives.

The current global situation has changed the dynamics of refugee experience. Large numbers of refugees are internally displaced, residing in countries that continue to suffer instability, with few resources for health care and other basic necessities and no opportunity to rebuild their lives and communities. This prolongation of the liminal state of being uprooted also occurs for those who migrate because they may wait long periods to be granted official refugee status and achieve citizenship rights. Others find themselves with no legal status at all, living in the interstices of societies without services, support, or protection. These forms of marginality and exclusion add to the burden of illness in refugee populations and contribute to persistent health problems.

The health of refugees reflects the illnesses endemic to their countries of origin and those they are exposed to on their way to asylum. To these are added specific problems that arise from the violent events that spur migration, compounded by the psychological distress created by prolonged uncertainty about the ultimate fate of self and loved ones. Refugees suffer multiple losses and challenges to their psychological integrity, all of which are likely to have profound implications for their health. As Derrick Silove has pointed out, exposure to massive human rights violations like torture, violent persecution, and genocide has effects that go far beyond the creation of fear and stress syndromes to include disruptions of attachment and security, interpersonal trust, and belief in a just and meaningful world. Failing to address these broader dimensions of refugee health from the start may lead to far greater problems down the line.

As a result of policies of deterrence, refugee claimants are made to wait for long periods uncertain about the outcome of their claim and subject to capricious treatment or even confinement under circumstances that test the limits of human resilience—all this while fearing for the safety and survival of loved ones left behind whom they hope to rescue once they gain a foothold in a safe place. The refugee determination process itself may be traumatic when adjudicators see their role as aggressively challenging the claims of people who are in a fragile and precarious position.

Although much attention is focused on refugee trauma and on the initial period of migration, when the person is formally an asylum seeker, the refugee trajectory is much longer, extending years into the future. We need to take the long view, beyond the urgency of the period of flight to consider the adaptation of refugees over time. In his ten-year follow-up study of South-East Asian refugees to Vancouver, Morton Beiser has shown clearly how the response of the host society is one of the overriding determinants of outcome. People seeking refuge who find a welcoming society in which they are able to find meaningful work, commensurate with their skills and talents, and maintain some continuity with their own culture, fare better than those who experience limited opportunities and pressure to abandon their core values and traditions.

As Pascale Allotey notes in her introductory chapter, 'Australia presents an interesting case study in this area as it grapples with paradoxes of multiculturalism, human rights obligations, and humanitarianism alongside harsh policies of state sovereignty and border protection'. Indeed, Australia is an important example for the rest of the world in several respects. It is a country of immigration, which is made up largely of settlers, many of whom found refuge from difficult situations in their countries of origin. This should confer a moral kinship between Australian citizens and newcomers who seek safety for their families and themselves. The cultural diversity that is woven into the fabric of Australian society should also promote awareness of the importance of cultural identity and continuity among refugees. Finally, Australia is wealthy country with highly developed infrastructure and health services and so has the resources to respond to the needs of refugees both at home and abroad. This response can provide a model of 'best practice' for other countries or an excuse for them to turn away. Of course, the dilemma of responding to refugees is not just a burden carried by the developed world, it is a problem for the most resource-poor and stressed regions of the world where most refugees reside.

Refugees share common predicaments but come from diverse cultural backgrounds. The field of refugee health must tackle questions of cultural diversity both in health care delivery and in social integration. The strangers at the gate are like us in their humanity and their basic needs for health, but they also are different in their ways of thinking about health, their hierarchies of values, and visions of the good life. Far from being a threat to our societies, they represent an opportunity for healthy confrontation with alternative ways of being.

Discussion of the health of refugees necessarily is rooted in consideration of humanitarian and human rights issues for it is this moral concern that creates the whole category of refugee. But this discussion tends to put the focus on the refugee as 'other' rather than on ourselves. The situation of refugees has implications for receiving societies. How we treat strangers in desperate need is a mark of our individual humanity, and of the values that define our society.

The response to refugees depends on moral imagination and political will. Imagination is needed in health care not only to respond in a humane and empathic way to the plight of individual refugees, but more broadly to develop creative responses in health care systems at home and abroad. This will support equitable access to care and help prevent the acute stress of forced migration from leading to chronic problems. Addressing the health needs of refugees can also have more far reaching effects, raising awareness of global disparities in health, wealth and power that fuel the conflicts that make people flee for their lives in the first place.

This book is unique in bringing together the methods and perspectives of public health, medicine, and human rights to address the health of refugees. The contributors give equal weight to quantitative and qualitative research, and to the voices of refugees themselves, expressed through their narratives. This is a crucial addition to the usual presentations of data, which may fail to capture the texture of experience. There is an ethical 'rigour' involved in listening closely and participating in people's lives long enough to get a clear sense of their predicament and priorities.

Indeed, the lessons learned from the narratives of refugees are crucial to ground our interventions. Listening closely to others, we recognise ourselves and with that comes the awareness that any of us might find ourselves in a similar quandary—fleeing for our lives, searching for a place that upholds human rights and allows us the dignity of moral action. As George Steiner once put it, 'Morality must always have its bags packed'.

Laurence J. Kirmayer
McGill University

Contents

List of figures and tables

List of abbreviations

ABS	Australian Bureau of Statistics
ALNAP	Active Learning Network on Accountability and Performance
AMEP	Adult Migration Education Program
ANCORW	Australian National Committee on Refugee Women
CAT	Convention Against Torture
CDNANZ	Communicable Diseases Network Australia and New Zealand
CEDAW	Convention on the Elimination of all forms of Discrimination Against Women
CHE	complex humanitarian emergency
CHW	community health worker
CPE	complex political emergency
CRC	Convention on the Rights of the Child
CRR	Centre for Refugee Research
DHAC	Department of Health and Aged Care
DIMIA	Department of Immigration and Multicultural and Indigenous Affairs
DOD	Department of Defence
DOH	Department of Health
ELR	Exceptional Leave to Remain
FARREP	Family and Reproductive Rights Education Program
HA	Health Authority
HSA	Health Services Australia
HAZ	Health Action Zone
HO	Home Office
HREOC	Human Rights and Equal Opportunity Commission
ICCPR	International Covenant on Civil and Political Rights
ICESCR	International Covenant on Economic, Social and Cultural Rights
ICRC	International Committee of the Red Cross
IDP	internally displaced person

IMF	International Monetary Fund
JSCSI	Joint Standing Committee on Social Issues (Australia)
MRC	Migrant Resource Centre
NFSSTT	National Forum of Services for Survivors of Torture and Trauma
NGO	Non-Governmental Organisation
NHMRC	National Health and Medical Research Council
PHLS	Public Health Laboratory Service
PTSD	post-traumatic stress disorder
SAC	Special Assistance Category
SAME	Sahel Africa and the Middle East
SHP	Special Humanitarian Program
STARTTS	Service for the Treatment and Rehabilitation of Torture and Trauma Survivors
STD	Sexually Transmitted Disease
STI	Sexually Transmissible Infection
TBA	traditional birth attendant
THS	Territory Health Services
TPV	Temporary Protection Visa
UDHR	Universal Declaration of Human Rights
UN	United Nations
UNAMET	United Nations Mission in East Timor
UNDP	United Nations Development Programme
UNHCR	United Nations High Commissioner for Refugees
UNRWA	United Nations Relief and Works Agency
VFST	Victorian Foundation for Survivors of Torture
WCH	women and children's health
WHO	World Health Organisation

Contributors

Pascale Allotey is a senior public health researcher with a background in medical anthropology and epidemiology. She has special interests in the health effects of social marginalisation (particularly as it is experienced by refugees), gender, and tropical health. She is a Senior Research Fellow at the Key Centre for Women's Health in Society at the University of Melbourne and a recipient of a prestigious Victorian Health Promotion Public Health Fellowship to undertake a program of research in the health of refugees and asylum seekers.

Astier M. Almedom (D.Phil.) is the Henry R. Luce Professor in Science and Humanitarianism at Tufts University, Department of Biology and the Gerald and Dorothy Friedman School of Nutrition Science and Policy, Boston, USA. She has both academic and practitioner insights, having worked in the London School of Hygiene and Tropical Medicine, where she lectured in medical anthropology, and the UK government National Health Service (NHS) senior management, where she served as Research and Evaluation Manager for Lambeth, Southwark, and Lewisham Health Action Zone, prior to joining Tufts University. Dr Almedom was educated at Oxford University: BA (Hons) in Human Sciences (1986) and D.Phil., in Biological Anthropology (1991).

Fatima Alvarez-Castillo is a Professor of Social Sciences at the University of the Philippines, teaching research methods, political economy and health anthropology. She is an academician and advocate. She works with non-governmental organisations and communities in advocating for social justice and respect for human rights. In her research she tries to build on methods that contribute to making researchers more ethical and participants more empowered. Among her published works are pieces on ethics and research, peasant consciousness and armed struggle, and community experience in empowerment.

Linda Bartolomei is the Senior Research Associate at the Centre for Refugee Research at the University of New South Wales and is the immediate past chair of the Australian National Committee on Refugee Women (ANCORW). She has represented ANCORW at several recent international United Nations meetings including: the Commission on the Status of Women, 2000; Beijing Plus Five; and the June 2000 Prepcom for the International Criminal Court. She is currently undertaking her PhD examining the impact of recent developments within International Law, policy and practice in addressing sexual violence experienced by refugee women and children.

Beverley-Ann Biggs is an infectious diseases physician with the Victorian Infectious Diseases Service, Royal Melbourne Hospital. She provides clinical care to immigrants and refugees in this setting and has a special interest in parasitic diseases. She is a senior lecturer at the University of Melbourne and has been involved in several research projects in African and Asian communities in Melbourne, and is the program director for an international health program that is working to strengthen immunisation programs in countries in the Mekong region.

Margaret Cunningham (MSW, Churchill Fellow) established the first funded Australian service for the treatment and rehabilitation of torture survivors. In this role she facilitated the development of torture and trauma services in each state of Australia and in New Zealand. She represented Australia on international committees on the care of torture survivors. She is a conjoint lecturer in the Faculty of Medicine at the University of New South Wales and was chair of the faculty's ethics and human rights group. She has international publications in relation to health service development and torture survivors, and has studied on scholarship at the Francoise Bagnoud Centre for Health and Human Rights at Harvard University, USA. She is currently employed at General Practice Education Australia and conducts a private consultancy in service development, design, and review of multicultural health services, and supervision of refugee workers in relation to their clinical practice, group work, and managing the context of their work environments.

Cathryn Finney Lamb was the research officer for the New South Wales Refugee Health Service at the time of writing this chapter. Prior to commencing there, she obtained a Masters in Public Health and had ten years experience in research in multicultural health. During this time she has conducted qualitative and quantitative research on health status, cultural and social determinants of health, and the effectiveness and appropriateness of health services and programs for immigrant populations.

Rachael Gosling worked as an advice worker and trainer for a number of refugee organisations in the voluntary sector in the UK, after obtaining a postgraduate diploma in refugee studies from Oxford University in 1995. She has undertaken research in Zambia and the Czech Republic on refugee issues. She spent two years coordinating the Health Action Zone Young Refugee Project in Lambeth, Southwark, and Lewisham, the first six months of which was dedicated to carrying out the research discussed in this book. She is currently working as a public health associate in Merseyside and Cheshire.

Ainslie Hannan has been the coordinator of the Ecumenical Migration Centre of the Brotherhood of St Laurence in Melbourne since February 2000. Prior to this she worked in settlement planning, social research, community health, housing, and family services. She has formal qualifications in social science, social work, management and social policy. Informing her practice is the belief in people's compassion, good will, and resilience. Until 2001 she chaired the Women's Health Centre and is the current chair of the Ministerial Northern Regional Youth Committee.

Bronwen Harvey is a medical adviser in the Commonwealth Department of Health and Ageing. Her clinical experience has been in general practice, child health and rehabilitation, and aged care. Within the department she has worked in the areas of public health, aged care, and general practice policy. She was a member of the departmental team that had responsibility for the health aspects of Operation Safe Haven.

Ida Kaplan is the direct services coordinator at the Victorian Foundation for Survivors of Torture (VFST), which principally involves overseeing client services, supervising all counselling work, and developing and delivering training programs. Her professional background is clinical psychology. The foundation services are aimed at enhancing recovery for adult, adolescent, and child refugees, and working collaboratively with agencies from a variety of sectors to meet client needs. She has had a long-time commitment to human rights and as part of the management team at VFST, contributing to systemic advocacy for survivors of human rights violations.

Laurence Kirmayer is a Professor of Psychiatry and Director of the Division of Social and Transcultural Psychiatry at McGill University, Canada. His background is in cultural psychiatry. He has published widely on issues concerning culture and psychiatric diagnosis, depression, and anxiety. He is particularly interested in psychiatric and cognitive enhancement and questions involving cross-cultural psychiatry.

Susan Kneebone is an Associate Professor in the Law Faculty, Monash University, where she works closely with the Castan Centre for Human Rights Law. Susan teaches administrative law and international refugee law and practice. She has published several articles on procedures for refugee status determination and on Australian refugee law issues. She has also made submissions to Senate and other inquiries into associated issues and is currently working on a large research project on comparative procedures for refugee status determination. In August 2002 she gave evidence to the Australian Senate's Legal and Constitutional References Committee's inquiry into migration zone excision. Susan is the editor of The Refugee Convention 50 Years On: Globalisation and International Law (Ashgate 2003) which is a collection of essays from a workshop she organised in June 2001.

Celia McMichael was awarded a Masters in Anthropology and Development at the University of Edinburgh in 1998. She has just completed a PhD at the Key Centre for Women's Health, School of Population Health, the University of Melbourne. Celia's research interests focus on community and emotional well-being among Somali women in Melbourne, and she is currently carrying out research around these issues for her doctoral thesis. Since April 2000 Celia has also been working at the Migrant Resource Centre North East in Melbourne, particularly with women from Somalia.

Professor Lenore Manderson is an inaugural Australia Research Council Federation Fellow at the Key Centre for Women's Health in Society, the University of Melbourne. She was previously Professor of Women's Health and Director of the Centre, and prior to that, from 1988 to 1998, she was Professor of Tropical Health at the University of Queensland. Lenore is a Fellow of the Academy of Social Sciences in Australia and is a member of the Executive of the Academy. She is President of the International Association for Study of Sexuality, Culture, and Society. She has several publications and a sustained research interest in the health of women in voluntary immigrant, refugee, and indigenous communities.

Peter Mares is a journalist with Radio Australia's *Asia Pacific* program and a visiting fellow at the Institute for Social Research at Swinburne University of Technology in Melbourne. He is the author of *Borderline: Australia's response to refugees and asylum seekers in the wake of the Tampa* (UNSW Press, Sydney 2002).

Professor Rob Moodie graduated in medicine from the University of Melbourne in 1976 and later trained in Tropical Medicine at Paris University, and Public Health at Harvard University. Professor Moodie is currently the Chief Executive Officer of VicHealth, an organisation that has a keen interest in promoting the health of marginalised populations and fostering community support towards population health and well-being. He has professorial appointments in public health at Melbourne and Monash Universities.

Eileen Pittaway is the Director of the Centre of Refugee Research University of New South Wales, Sydney, and a member of the Asian Women's Human Rights Council. She has been working in the field of refugee policy for twenty-five years, focusing mainly on the needs of refugee women and their children. She represented one of International non-governmental organisations who successfully lobbied at the United Nations for recognition of rape in conflict situations as a war crime. Her research interests include the relationship between civil society and the United Nations.

Susan A. Skull is a public health physician, epidemiologist, and paediatrician working as Deputy Director of the Clinical Epidemiology and Biostatistics Unit of the Royal Children's Hospital. She is also a senior lecturer with the Department of Paediatrics at the University of Melbourne. She has been involved in establishing clinical services for immigrants and refugees, and research projects in conjunction with refugee communities in Melbourne. She is working with the Department of Human Services, Victoria and others to develop a model of immigrant health service delivery in Victoria, focusing on public health service infrastructure, education of health professionals and the community, and research.

Derrick Silove (FRANZCP, MD) is a Professor of Psychiatry at the University of New South Wales and Director of the Psychiatry Research and Teaching Unit at Liverpool Hospital. He is a board member, past chair and consulting psychiatrist at STARTTS, the New South Wales torture and trauma service for refugees. He directs PRADET, the Psychosocial Recovery and Development program in East Timor.

Dr Mitchell Smith is a public health physician who is currently Director of the New South Wales Refugee Health Service. His involvement with refugees began in 1988 teaching Afghan medics in northern Pakistan. He then worked in Hong Kong for Médecins sans Frontières on a health care program for Vietnamese boat people. During Operation Safe Haven in 1999 he acted as medical coordinator for South Western Sydney Area Health Service, helping oversee health services for evacuees at the East Hills Reception Centre and Safe Haven, on the outskirts of Sydney.

Dr Michael J. Toole is a medical epidemiologist and public health physician with special interests in refugees and humanitarian emergencies, HIV/AIDS prevention and care, nutrition, and communicable disease control. He is currently Head of the Centre for International Health of the Burnet Institute for Medical Research and Public Health in Melbourne. He is also Associate Professor in the Department of Epidemiology and Preventive Medicine at Melbourne's Monash University. He is vice-president of Médecins sans Frontières, Australia.

Kim Webster has worked extensively in the areas of family violence, women's health, and refugee health and settlement. As a Victorian Government policy officer she drafted *Criminal Assault in the Home: Social and Legal Responses to Domestic Violence*, and contributed to the development of women's health policy and services in Victoria. She has also drafted a number of publications and reports on behalf of women's health and refugee non-government and consumer advocacy groups. Kim currently works at the Victorian Foundation for Survivors of Torture where her publications include the *Refugee Health and General Practice Handbook* and *Refugee Resettlement: An International Handbook to Guide Reception and Integration*, produced on behalf of the United Nations High Commissioner for Refugees (UNHCR).

Anthony Zwi was born in South Africa where he also studied medicine, occupational health, and tropical medicine. He left South Africa to train in public health and epidemiology in the United Kingdom, and subsequently spent ten years in the Health Policy Unit at the London School of Hygiene and Tropical Medicine. In April 2001 he was appointed Professor and Head of the School of Public Health and Community Medicine at the University of New South Wales. His interests relate to conflict and health, international health policy, humanitarian health policy, and policy accountability. He has a particular interest in how individuals and systems survive adversity. He has published widely and is keen to utilise the potential of the World Wide Web and new technologies more generally, to stimulate debate and critique about changing global health policies. He is interested in how organisations learn and is interested in promoting and supporting reflective organisations and practitioners. He has worked with non-governmental organisations on Writing, Reflection and Policy (WRAP) workshops, with a view to producing material and experience that can be placed in the public domain where it can be debated and critiqued.

Introduction

Asylum seekers are people who have been forced to flee from their homes and countries of origin to seek refuge elsewhere for reasons that may involve the difference between life and death. When their plight is officially recognised through processes that have been set up by the United Nations and the countries that offer temporary or permanent refuge, the 'label' is changed from asylum seeker to refugee. The response of the international community; a) to the situations that create refugees and b) to the obligation to protect people who no longer enjoy the protection of their own governments and are seeking asylum or refuge, is tempered by the complexities of political interests, immigration policies and border sovereignty. Often lost in these complexities are the specific health needs of this group whose vulnerabilities are created by a combination of the outcomes of conflict, displacement, poverty, natural disasters and/or violations of their human rights. Also lost is the heterogeneity of this population; the significant differences created by gender, culture, socio-economic status, and circumstances that provide the context for short and long-term health outcomes in all populations.

Refugee health, while clearly under the rubric of public health, often has a very specific meaning depending on the context in which it is being used. In humanitarian emergencies, it usually refers to the acute management of the health issues involved in massive population movements as a result of natural disasters or complex humanitarian crises created by conflict and war. In the context of displacement, a situation that often occurs within the national borders of the affected population, it refers to public health management to control the spread of infectious diseases that are rife in the conditions created by poor hygiene, over-crowding and lack of health service infrastructure. In the process of resettlement to third countries, refugee health involves rigorous health screening and assessments to identify exotic communicable diseases that might threaten the public health of host nations and following resettlement it refers to the management of health and health services to control the potential for the marginalisation of minority resettled populations, spanning the provision of cultural competencies for health service staff to addressing the specific physical and mental needs of torture and trauma survivors.

Current public health discourse has expanded the role of public health researchers and practitioners to include a more central role in advocacy to ensure a more equitable distribution of the resources that enable health and access to health care particularly to the marginalised and vulnerable. There is a greater imperative for involvement in the political, economic, and social issues that shape a rapidly globalising world with repercussions on increasing disparities in health and wealth, the potential for conflict and the core issues that result in the creation of displaced people and refugees. The human rights framework that highlights the importance of a multi-disciplinary focus currently provides some tools with which advocacy in this area can be negotiated.

This book attempts to draw together what can essentially be described as the continuum of refugee health issues tracing the health consequences on individuals and populations from situations of conflict through the process of resettlement in countries other than their countries of origin. The collection of papers brings together a broad range of disciplines including human rights and humanitarian law, journalism, public health research and practice as well as social work and community development, to provide a holistic perspective on the health of refugees and asylum seekers. In compiling these papers, the aim is to highlight the complexity of factors that influence the health of refugees and asylum seekers and the development of the health policies concerning this vulnerable group. In addition, the collection also provides a resource that contributes to the public debate in this increasingly important area of public health.

The focus of the research and practice described in the text is largely on Australia. While it does not have the proximity and refugee crises of nations closer to regions of conflict, Australia presents an interesting case study in this area as it grapples with what have become paradoxes of multiculturalism, human rights obligations and humanitarianism on the one hand and policies of state sovereignty and border protection on the other.

Outline of the book

The book is divided into four parts. Part one provides the background information establishing the international contexts of the current refugee situation. Kneebone and Allotey explain the human rights and humanitarian framework on which international protection of refugees is based in chapter one. The global context for refugee health is laid out by Zwi and Castillo in chapter two, bringing 'the big picture into focus' by discussing globalisation as the backdrop to the current situation on conflict, complex humanitarian and political emergencies that have resulted in chronic mass movements of people and an escalating refugee crisis. In chapter three, Toole discusses the public health concerns that arise from working with refugees internationally, drawing on several years of experience with Médecins sans Frontières and the Centers for Disease Control and Prevention in Atlanta, USA.

In part two a series of papers detail the specific health issues of refugees during resettlement. In chapter four, Biggs and Skull present data from their work with the infectious diseases unit of a hospital in Melbourne, Australia, that provides specialised services and screening to refugee groups. They also highlight some of the problems faced by refugees in interacting with health services. Silove, in chapter five, discusses the mental health of refugees, particularly of asylum seekers in detention and begins to highlight some of the long-term implications of what he describes as gross violations of their human rights. Pittaway and Bartolomei also discuss mental health associated with detention but focus specifically on children within the broader framework of the Convention on the Rights of the Child in chapter six. Kaplan and Webster raise the important gender issues by discussing the refugee experience and mental health of refugee women in chapter seven. They also highlight some specific strategies for promoting the health of refugee women.

Part three of the book is a discussion of the health service delivery to refugees and asylum seekers. In chapter eight, Finney Lamb and Cunningham present a comprehensive review of the models of service delivery and develop the debate on the advantages and disadvantages of providing specialised services to refugees versus broadening the scope and expertise of the mainstream health services to cater for minority groups. Operation Safe Haven, described by Smith and Harvey in chapter nine was a program that involved multi-sectoral collaboration to temporarily host several thousand evacuees from Kosovo and East Timor in Australia. The chapter highlights the difficulties in providing health care similar to the responses of the international community in emergency situations in developing countries, but within a nation that is well-off by most standards. In chapter ten Hannan presents an essay that describes service delivery for holders of the newly legislated Temporary Protection Visas for asylum seekers, drawing on a personal journal and experiences establishing Melbourne's first funded program for this minority group.

Public health research with refugee communities in resettlement countries frequently presents methodological challenges. The nature of the population makes them difficult to access and sample and therefore to obtain generalisable findings. These methodological issues are particularly pertinent in public health because of the dominant focus on epidemiological design and this highlights an important need to develop this area of public health research. The chapters in part four highlight a number of research projects based largely on qualitative and ethnographic designs. They highlight the importance of the research relationship with refugees and the need to address the dearth of evidence in this area without over researching the population. Almedom and Gosling, in chapter eleven, present the findings of an action research project in the UK and stress the importance of evaluation and the development of best practice models through rigorous research and community involvement. McMichael describes the research process she undertook as an ethnographer working with a minority population of 'vulnerable yet resilient' Somali women in chapter twelve and Allotey and Manderson emphasise the ethical issues and obligations of public health researchers in working with refugee groups in chapter thirteen.

Chapter fourteen, written by Mares and Allotey describes the role of the media in shaping public policy in refugee health. The advocacy role of public health researchers and practitioners in this area is largely dependent on the political climate, and the response of communities and the media play a central role in this relationship. Some suggestions are proposed about how the media can be employed to enhance public health advocacy in this area.

I would like to express my sincere thanks to all the contributors for generously giving their time to complete the manuscript. Lenore Manderson has been a very supportive mentor and insisted that I could do this and I am sincerely grateful for her confidence in me. Sandy Gifford, Anthony Zwi, and Helen Potts have been invaluable sounding boards. I would also like to acknowledge Heather Fawcett for taking a chance on me and Debra James for her incredible support through the editing process. Finally, I would like to thank Daniel for providing the 'nourishment for the growth of the tall poppy'.

Pascale Allotey

Refugee Health, Humanitarianism, and Human Rights

Susan Kneebone and Pascale Allotey

Everyone has the right to seek and enjoy in other countries asylum from persecution

Article 14, Universal Declaration of Human Rights

Introduction

This chapter presents a broad overview of issues relating to refugees and their health in the light of the applicable human rights framework. We consider both the international framework and the way that it has been translated into Australian law to give a context for understanding the health implications.

The prime instrument is the 1951 Convention Relating to the Status of Refugees[1] (the Refugee Convention), which was a global response that recognised the vulnerability and the need for protection of large numbers of people fleeing from Nazi Germany and communist Russia in post World War II. Article IA of the Refugee Convention defines a refugee as a person who has a:

> well-founded fear of being persecuted for reasons of race, religion, nationality, membership of a particular social group or political opinion, is outside the country of his nationality and is unable, or owing to such fear, is unwilling to avail himself of the protection of that country; or who, not having a national-ity and being outside the country of his former habitual residence, is unable or, owing to such fear, is unwilling to return to it.

Fifty years on, the situations that result in mass displacement and the creation of refugees are highly complex and have given rise to extensive debates about the reach of the refugee definition in the Refugee Convention, which requires an asylum seeker to have crossed the border of his or her country in order to gain refugee status. The current reality is that while there are potentially 12 million convention refugees worldwide, by far the greater number of persons in refugee-like situations, who are in need of protection from persecution, are contained within the borders of their country and are therefore not covered by the Refugee Convention. It has been estimated that the number of such internally displaced persons (IDPs) totalled 25 million as at the end of 2001.[2] Of this figure, the bulk, (13.5 million) were in Africa.

The causes of this mass displacement can be broadly described as arising from situations affecting large civilian populations involving a combination of factors including war or civil unrest, famine, and population displacement and resulting in significant excess mortality (Burkholder & Toole 1995). These situations can be defined as complex humanitarian emergencies (CHEs). More specifically, complex political emergencies (CPEs) focus on situations that involve violent conflict and highlight the political contribution to the crisis (Goodhand & Hulme 1999). CPEs typically occur across state boundaries, have political antecedents relating to competition for power and resources, are protracted in duration, are embedded in existing social, political, economic, and cultural structures and are often characterised by 'predatory' social domination (Goodhand & Hulme 1999). CPEs reflect a fundamental conceptual shift in the nature of war from an involvement between states, military capacities and strategies to the targeting of civilians. There has been an increase from 5 per cent civilian casualties in World War I to figures in excess of 80 per cent of civilian casualties in conflicts over the last five years (Benjamin 2001).

As a result of mass displacements, people affected by CPEs are vulnerable, politically and socially marginalised and lack access to basic food, shelter and often health and social services. Within refugee camps they may be subject to violence, neglect and violation of their human rights. Vulnerability can continue post-conflict, with the favourable outcome being a return to a stable social and political environment. This may be through repatriation to the country of origin when the stability returns, relocation to a neighbouring country or resettlement in a third, usually an industrialised Western country.

By its very nature, the protection of asylum seekers and refugees is a humanitarian issue, recognising the vulnerability of particular populations and the need to provide assistance. It is also an international human rights issue because of the inability or reluctance of governments to enforce laws to protect the basic human rights of the vulnerable.

Public health practitioners have a responsibility to ensure that policies exist to maximise health and well-being as well as equity of access to health care and health related services for the most vulnerable groups within the population. The constitution of the World Health Organisation, in 1946, recognised the importance of the enjoyment of the highest attainable standard of health as a fundamental human right. This was further reflected in the Alma Ata Declaration on Primary Health Care in 1978. However, it has only been in the last decade that the links between health and human rights have been increasingly acknowledged, growing out of the recognition of the value of the application of international law to address the protection of human rights and health care for marginalised populations, initially, with people living with HIV/AIDS (Gruskin & Tarantola 2002). The use of the human rights framework to advocate for the health and health care of individuals and populations more broadly has since become critical in public health to address increasing health inequalities and inequitable access to care in a rapidly changing climate of globalisation, health transition, and the spread of new and re-emerging communicable diseases. It provides an ideal benchmark for the assessment of the health of refugees and asylum seekers; a population that arguably presents one of the most significant human rights challenges that confront public health today (Dualeh & Paul 2002). It also enables us to acknowledge the rights of individuals as unique in their circumstances and context; a frequent oversight when all categories of asylum seekers and refugees are homogenised into a single amorphous group of non-citizens.

An historical perspective

The history of the twentieth century is marked by its refugee crises. Indeed until the beginning of that century, and for some time after, nations prided themselves on their humanitarian approach to asylum seekers, whose addition to the community was seen as an enhancement to its reputation. In response to catastrophic events created by the breakdown of the old European empires, various treaties from the 1920s onwards began to define the rights of particular categories of refugees to seek asylum in specific situations, such as the Armenian refugees and persons of Russian origin (Fortin 2001). The first international agreements defined a refugee as a person who no longer enjoyed the protection of their government and had not acquired another nationality. The first formal refugee-specific organisation set up after the formation of the United Nations (UN) was the United Nations Relief and Works Agency (UNRWA) for Palestinian Refugees, mandated by a UN Security Council resolution in 1949. The UNRWA has been responsible for delivering basic services including food, shelter, health, and education to Palestinian refugees since 1950 and given the continuing unrest in the region, its mandate continues to be renewed by the UN General Assembly.

The 1951 Refugee Convention, administered through the United Nations High Commissioner for Refugees (UNHCR), differed from its predecessors in providing a generalised and individualised definition of a refugee. The key to the definition is proof of a 'well-founded fear of being persecuted' for the reasons set out in the convention. In 1951 the convention was intended to deal with people fleeing actual physical persecution as well as those fleeing for ideological reasons. Its meaning is clearly and intentionally broad. The removal of the reference to the time limitation of 1951 by the 1967 Protocol showed that it was intended to be a flexible document. Article 33 of the Refugee Convention contains what is often said to be the underlying principle of the convention. This is the *non-refoulement* provision, which imposes an obligation on a Contracting state not to return *(refoule)* a person to the frontiers of a territory where his life or freedom would be threatened for any one of the reasons set out in the refugee definition in Article 1A (UNHCR 1951, 1967).

The Refugee Convention is part of a range of international instruments or agreements that provide for human rights protection. Its provisions against persecution are complemented by the Universal Declaration of Human Rights (UDHR), Article 14 (the 'right of flight' provision stated as the opening quote of the chapter),[3] the Convention Against Torture and other Cruel or Degrading Treatment or Punishment (CAT) discussed below, and the International Covenant on Civil and Political Rights (ICCPR). For example, Article 2 contains an undertaking to respect the rights of individuals present within a territory, without 'distinction of any kind'.[4] This is arguably the basis upon which international law requires states to protect foreign individuals, in contrast to the exclusionary notion of protection based upon allegiance and corresponding sovereignty. Article 7 states that 'No one shall be subjected to torture or to cruel, inhuman or degrading treatment'. Other guarantees in the Refugee Convention (such as the right to work, education, and travel documents) are consistent with general human rights provisions. For example, UDHR Article 13 contains the right to freedom of movement, Article 23 the right of *everyone* to work, Article 25 states that everyone has the right to a standard of living adequate for health and well-being and Article 26 states the right to education.

The Refugee Convention does not define the meaning of persecution, but Articles 31 and 33 which refer to the threat to 'life or freedom' suggest that its core meaning includes deprivation of life or physical freedom (Goodwin-Gill 1996). This is consistent with CAT, which defines 'torture' as any act by which 'severe pain or suffering, whether physical or mental, is intentionally inflicted on a person'. The deprivation of life or physical freedom can be classified as the most fundamental of the basic human rights, which are recognised by international instruments. To this could be added freedom from torture or slavery, freedom of thought, religion, conscience, and the right to recognition as a person in law. Generally the courts both internationally and in Australia have recognised as acts of 'persecution' both physical and psychological torture as well as discrimination against an individual which amounts to a serious breach of a human right. For example, it has been recognised that women who are forced to leave their homes because their lives are at risk as a result of false accusations of adultery are at risk of persecution. Recently the High Court of Australia recognised that a 'black child' (a child born outside of China's one child policy) who would be denied basic rights to education and living standards was at risk of persecution if returned to China. But an Indian woman divorcee who had undergone a voluntary abortion and who claimed that she would be ostracised and similarly deprived in her traditional society was not given protection as a refugee. Generally in assessing whether there is a 'well-founded fear of being persecuted', the courts distinguish between persecution, which affects the basic human right to life or physical freedom, and mere hardship or discrimination of a social or economic nature.

The Refugee Convention definition in Article 1A set out above concentrates upon a person's civil or political status and has been linked more to the ICCPR. In Australia the ICCPR has been incorporated into federal law through annexing it to the Human Rights and Equal Opportunities Commission (HREOC) Act providing support for the politicisation of refugee issues. However, some refugee advocates have argued for a broader application of the definition of persecution to include other potentially life-threatening events such as those covered within the International Covenant on Economic, Social and Cultural Rights (ICESCR), which while ratified, has not been incorporated into legislation in countries such as Australia and is generally regarded as aspirational rather than dealing with rights per se. Significantly, in Article 2:3 of ICESCR, specific reference is made to the exception to which the economic rights of non-nationals may not be guaranteed and that occurs only within developing countries where there is economic hardship. The ICESCR is important in this area however, because it provides support for cases such as gender related persecution (Copelon 2000; Kelley 2001). The case of Togolese Fauziya Kasinga receiving asylum in the US in 1996 based on her fear of female genital mutilation provided an opportunity to set precedents in this.

In becoming signatories to the various human rights conventions, governments assume the responsibility and obligation to ensure that every individual enjoys the rights stated in the particular instrument. In addition, the government has to:

- respect and may not directly violate the rights of individuals which includes making arbitrary decisions to withhold care;
- protect rights and prevent violations by non-state actors and provide redress for when violations occur; and
- fulfil rights by taking all appropriate measures to incrementally allocate sufficient resources to meet the public health needs of communities within its borders.

Implementation of the Refugee Convention

We take the example of Australia to show how the obligations as a signatory to the Refugee Convention may be implemented in national law. The purpose of this discussion is to show how facets of the system have implications for the health of refugees.

Australia's international obligation to refugees is administered by the Department of Immigration and Multicultural and Indigenous Affairs (DIMIA) under the Humanitarian Program. Since 1996 the government has maintained a program of 12,000 places per annum. This quota comprises two components. The onshore component offers protection to non-citizens who arrive on Australian shores with or without a valid visa and claim asylum (asylum seekers). To qualify for protection, this category of person needs to meet the high standard of the definition of a 'refugee' in the 1951 Refugee Convention. This is incorporated into the Migration Act (1958). There is a nominal quota of 2000 places for this category although in recent years due to the demand for places this number has been exceeded. For example in 2000–2001, 5577 onshore protection visas were granted (Australian Department of Immigration and Multicultural and Indigenous Affairs (DIMIA) 2001). The other part of the program, the 'offshore' component (with a nominal quota of 10,000 places) includes persons of concern, often in refugee camps who are identified and selected by the Australian Government for resettlement in conjunction with the UNHCR, the International Red Cross, and other humanitarian agencies.

The offshore resettlement program establishes a hierarchy, which in part reflects the seriousness of the circumstances of the refugees. Primarily, it includes persons who have been recognised as refugees by the UNHCR and are in need of resettlement (this is a refugee category with a nominal allocation of about 4000) (Australian Department of Immigration and Multicultural and Indigenous Affairs (DIMIA) 2001). These people have largely been living in exile in neighbouring states, in refugee camps or under UNHCR protection, in those countries where such facilities exist. Often they have existed in this temporary state of uncertainty for a number of years. Australia is one of the top three UNHCR resettlement countries. The top two are the USA and Canada who respectively take in about 72,500 and 13,500 persons per annum. The UNHCR resettles approximately 98,000 persons annually under this scheme. This is a small number in proportion to the total refugee problem (12 million). The slowness and uncertainty of this process is one of the reasons why asylum seekers often seek alternative options such as 'people smugglers' to seek asylum onshore.

The second category under the offshore component of the humanitarian program is the Special Humanitarian Program (SHP), of about 3000. This is for people who have suffered discrimination amounting to gross violations of human rights, including 'women at risk', and who have strong support from an Australian citizen or resident or community group in Australia (Manderson et al. 1998). Thirdly, included within this figure is a smaller number identified as within the Special Assistance Category (SAC). This is for persons who do not meet the criteria for the other categories but who nevertheless are in situations of discrimination, hardship, or displacement. They are usually proposed by a close relative in Australia. These latter categories require sponsoring communities to share the financial burden of the government's humanitarian program as state benefits to the latter categories are more restrictive.

Australia has long had a policy that is aimed at deterring onshore asylum seekers. Two manifestations of this are the mandatory detention system and the Temporary Protection Visa (TPV) system (see Hannan p. 156). The mandatory detention system was introduced with bipartisan support in 1992. Detention is permissible in international and human rights law and practice if it is deemed necessary for public health, public safety, security, and identification (United Nations High Commissioner for Refugees). However, indefinite detention, with no access to judicial review is not (Sidoti 2002). Prolonged detention is contrary to Article 31 of the Refugee Convention, which states that parties shall not impose penalties upon asylum seekers because of their illegal presence in a country. It has been argued that mandatory detention is arbitrary and in breach of Article 9 of the ICCPR. The Australian Government's detention policy includes controversially the detention of children which breaches many of the provisions of the Convention on the Rights of the Child (CRC) (see Pittaway and Bartolomei p. 83). In its 1998 report, *Those Who've Come Across the Seas: Detention of Unauthorised Arrivals*, the HREOC argued for an alternative model of detention. Despite similar recommendations from other groups the government has not acted to modify the mandatory detention policy, which unquestionably has profound health implications (discussed by Silove p. 72 and Pittaway and Bartolomei p. 87).

The second deterrent policy is the Temporary Protection Visa category (TPV) which was introduced in October 1999. This three-year visa may be available to non-citizens who arrive on Australian shores after that date without proper documentation. Prior to that, onshore asylum seekers who satisfied the Refugee Convention definition, were granted permanent protection visas. The TPV denies the holders a number of basic rights, such as re-entry to Australia. This appears to be in breach of the Refugee Convention Article 28 which states that 'Contracting States shall issue to refugees lawfully staying in their territory travel documents for the purpose of travel outside their territory unless compelling reasons of national security or public order otherwise require…'. The holders are also denied family unification. In late 2001 a tragedy occurred that involved the drowning of over 300 asylum seekers off the Indonesian coast. The Minister for Immigration Philip Ruddock refused to waive this condition to enable distraught TPV holders to identify the bodies of relatives. They have no right to the full range of settlement services and to welfare assistance (Corlett 2000). It is clear that this class of refugees holding TPVs is severely disadvantaged and that it has created a discriminated subclass with serious health problems (see also Hannan chapter).

In September 2001 the Australian Government introduced new legislation to deal with the processing of asylum seekers who seek to apply for protection under the Refugee Convention. The legislation was in response to the dramatic events of the MV *Tampa* crisis in Australia's northern waters in late August 2001 when the Australian Government refused to allow the captain of a Norwegian cargo ship, which had rescued a 'cargo' of 433 asylum seekers, to disembark them onto Christmas Island for processing as refugees (Mares 2001). A package of legislation established the 'Pacific Plan' pursuant to which most offshore Australian islands are no longer part of Australia's migration zone. Applications for protection visas cannot be made from those 'excised' territories. Other legislation empowers the Australian authorities to intercept boat arrivals and to remove them to detention processing facilities on various Pacific Islands (currently Nauru and Manus Island in New Guinea) which participate in 'the plan'. At the same time a new regime of visas was introduced. The legislation effectively means that arrivals who have been in transit in a country other than their country of origin cannot apply for permanent protection visas. The legislation also establishes an extended hierarchy of Temporary Protection Visas (TPVs) intended to deter persons from making secondary movements by travelling through safe countries.

As a result of the new legislation, two systems are currently operating for the processing of onshore arrivals. There are those who are processed offshore under the Pacific Plan, and those who are processed onshore under Australian law. In the case of the Pacific Plan, the processing is shared by the Australian Government, and the UNHCR. Applicants who are processed under the Pacific Plan have an internal right of review to a DIMIA officer, and can seek a remedy in the High Court. By contrast persons who apply onshore for the protection visas have a right of review to the Refugee Review Tribunal. From that decision either the minister or the applicant can seek judicial review, which is a limited type of appeal on questions of law, either from the Federal Court or the High Court. These processes can be very lengthy, and are uncertain in their outcome. As applicants are detained until the exhaustion of these processes, this has significant implications for mental health (see Silove).

The fairness of the procedures described is open to question. Recent decisions of the High Court (2000, 2001) and commentaries by observers of the system (Kneebone 2002) suggest that in many instances applicants do not receive a fair hearing. Although various human rights instruments assume that an asylum seeker has a right to a fair hearing, it is nowhere directly stated. Article 14 of the UDHR enshrines the basic right to seek asylum, Article 14 of the ICCPR states that all persons shall be entitled to a fair and public hearing by a competent and impartial tribunal, and Article 16 of the Refugee Convention states that a refugee shall have free access to the courts of law. The nearest statement of a right to a *fair* hearing is contained in the UNHCR handbook on procedures and criteria for determining refugee status. However, the Australian Government has recently legislated to remove the right to seek a remedy for an unfair decision.

Various reviews to determine whether Australia is in breach of its human rights obligations with regards to asylum seekers have been equivocal depending on who conducts them and it has never been clear that the government has felt any obligation to amend policies on the basis of the findings of these reviews (McMaster 2001; Sidoti 2002). Human rights experts have reported gross violations in several articles of the CROC, ICCPR, ICESCR, CAT and the Convention on the Elimination of all Forms of Racial Discrimination (Amnesty International Australia 1998; Bhagwati 2002). Somewhat alarmingly, an increasing global shift to conservative right-wing political ideals makes Australia a benchmark for countries, particularly in Europe, who are looking to replicate the policies to control the flow of asylum seekers into their countries (de Bousingen 2002; Lubbers & Scheepers 2001; Steiner 2000).

Health and rights of refugees

Everyone has the right to a standard of living adequate for the health and well-being of himself and his family, including food, clothing, housing and medical care and necessary social services, and the right to security in the event of unemployment, sickness, widowhood, old age or other lack of livelihood in circumstances beyond his control.

Article 25:1 UDHR

The States Parties to the present Covenant recognize the right of everyone to the enjoyment of the highest attainable standard of physical and mental health.

Article 12:1 ICESCR

Paragraph 1 of the General Comment 14 of the right to health contained within the ICESCR states that health is a fundamental human right indispensable for the exercise of other human rights (2000). Indeed it is difficult to imagine how health and well-being can be achieved with the neglect or violation of rights. People fleeing war-torn regions are often politically and socially marginalised and subject to violence and neglect or violation of many of their rights, including those relating to access to basic social services. In countries where they resettle if unable to return home, restrictive policies and community attitudes towards refugees in general and asylum seekers in particular may restrict access to services or present major barriers to utilisation (Jones 2000; Sales 2002). While the emphasis has thus far been on asylum seekers, there is evidence of widespread violations of human rights not only of refugees but of migrants more generally (Gerhart 1999; Morris 1998; Taran 2000). This is bound in the complexities of marginalisation, low status, inadequately regulated economic sectors, and competition for public goods such as health, welfare, and education.

In recognition of the potential for human rights violations of groups such as refugees and asylum seekers paragraph 34 of the General Comment on ICESCR (2000) that underlines legal obligations of the Covenant, states:

In particular, States are under the obligation to respect the right to health by, inter alia, refraining from denying or limiting equal access for all persons, including prisoners or detainees, minorities, asylum seekers and illegal immigrants, to preventive, curative and palliative health services; abstaining from enforcing discriminatory practices as a State policy...

The application of legal and human rights frameworks to promoting health and preventing disease has important advantages in that they provide the tools to support advocates in ensuring that governments meet their obligations towards the realisation of the rights to health of all people under its protection. As proponents of public health in general and advocates for the health and access to health care of populations that are marginalised in particular, public health professionals are uniquely placed to draw on the link between health and human rights. A disadvantage, which is evident in Australia, is the tendency for governments with a political agenda that may be at odds with humanitarian obligations, to capitalise on these frameworks either to institute the barest minimum required or to subject the obligations to restrictive interpretation.

Where economics, politics, and international law have failed, health can be used as a platform to promote positive media and political attention towards refugees and asylum seekers (Hargreaves 2001). Systematic investigation and documentation of the effects of conflict, displacement, resettlement, and refugee policies on the health of refugees and asylum seekers as well as on the host populations is vital to the assessment of the long-term implications of rapid global changes and movements of people.

Recommended readings

Chimni, B. (ed.) (2000) *International Refugee Law. A reader,* Sage Publications, New Delhi.

Gruskin, S. & Tarantola, D. (2002) Health and Human Rights, In Detels, R., McEwen, J., Beaglehole, R. & Tanaka, H. (eds) *Oxford Textbook of Public Health* vol. 1, Oxford University Press, Oxford, pp. 311–35.

Human Rights Watch (2001) Refugees, asylum seekers and internally displaced persons, 50 years on: what future for international refugee protection, *Human Rights Watch World Report 2001*, Human Rights Watch, New York, pp. 509–21.

Mann, J., Gruskin, S., Grodin, M.L. & Annas, G.J. (eds) (1999) *Health and Human Rights: A Reader*, Routledge, New York.

Steiner, H.J. & Alston, P. (2000) *International Human Rights in Context: Law, Politics, Morals*, Oxford University Press, Oxford.

Taran, P. (2000) Human rights of migrants: challenges of the new decade, *International Migration*, 38(6): 7–51.

References

Refugee Review Tribunal (2000) Ex parte Aala Canberra.

Minister for Immigration (2001) Ex parte Miah Canberra.

Amnesty International Australia (1998) *Australia, A Continuing Shame: The mandatory detention of asylum seekers*, Amnesty International Australia, Sydney.

Australia (1958) *Migration Act*, Commonwealth of Australia, Canberra.

Australian Department of Immigration and Multicultural and Indigenous Affairs (DIMIA) (2001) Fact Sheet 60, DIMIA, Canberra.

Benjamin, J.A. (2001) Conflict, post conflict and HIV AIDS—the gender connections. Women, War and HIV/AIDS: West Africa and the Great Lakes, In *World Bank, International Women's Day* World Bank, Washington DC.

Bhagwati, P. (2002) *Detention centres in Australia*, United Nations High Commissioner for Human Rights, Geneva.

Burkholder, B. & Toole, M. (1995) Evolution of complex disasters, *Lancet*, 346: 1012–15.

Committee on Economic, Social and Cultural Rights (2000) *The right to the highest attainable standard of health: CESCR General comment 14*, United Nations, Geneva.

Copelon, R. (2000) Gender Crimes as War Crimes: Integrating Crimes against Women into International Criminal Law, *McGill Law Journal*, 46: 217–40.

Corlett, D. (2000) Politics, Symbolism and the Asylum Seeker Issue, *UNSW Law Journal*, 23: 3.

de Bousingen, D.D. (2002) Health issues and the rise of Le Pen in France, *Lancet*, 359: 1673.

Dualeh, M. & Paul, S. (2002) Refugees and other displaced populations, In Detels, R., McEwen, J., Beaglehole, R. & Tanaka, H. (eds), *Oxford Textbook of Public Health* vol. 3, Oxford University Press, Oxford, pp. 1737–54.

Fortin, A. (2001) The Meaning of "Protection" in the Refugee Definition', *International Journal of Refugee Law,* 12(4): 548.

Gerhart, G. (1999) Prohibited persons: abuse of undocumented migrants, asylum seekers and refugees in South Africa, *Foreign Affairs*, 78(2): 159.

Global IDP Project (2002) *A Global Overview of Internal Displacement*, Norwegian Refugee Council, Geneva.

Goodhand, J. & Hulme, D. (1999) From wars to complex political emergencies: understanding conflict and peace-building in the new world disorder, *Third World Quarterly*, 20(1): 13–26.

Goodwin-Gill, G. (ed) (1996) *The Refugee in International Law*, Clarendon Press, Oxford, pp. 67–8.

Gruskin, S. & Tarantola, D. (2002) Health and Human Rights, In Detels, R., McEwen, J., Beaglehole, R. & Tanaka, H. (eds) *Oxford Textbook of Public Health*, vol. 1, Oxford University Press, Oxford, pp. 311–35.

Hargreaves, S. (2001) Refugees: 50 years on, *Lancet*, 357: 1384.

Jones, J. (2000) Asylum seekers in UK receive poor health care, *British Medical Journal*, 320(7248): 1492.

Kelley, N. (2001) The convention refugee definition and gender based persecution: a decade's progress, *International Journal of Refugee Law*, 13(4): 559–68.

Kneebone, S. (2002) Fairness in Tribunals—Issues Relating to the RRT and Bias In *Adelaide Legal Convention*, Adelaide.

Lubbers, M. & Scheepers, P. (2001) Explaining the trend in extreme right wing voting: Germany 1989–1998, *European Sociological Review*, 17(4): 431–49.

Manderson, L., Kelaher, M., Markovic, M. & McManus, K. (1998) A Woman without a Man is a Woman at Risk: Women at Risk in Australian Humanitarian Programs, *Journal of Refugee Studies*, 11(3): 267–83.

Mares, P. (2001) *Borderline,* UNSW Press, Sydney.

McMaster, D. (2001) *Asylum seekers. Australia's response to refugees*, Melbourne University Press, Melbourne.

Morris, A. (1998) Our fellow Africans make our lives hell—the lives of Congolese and Nigerians living in Johannesburg, *Ethnic and Racial Studies*, 21(6): 1116–36.

Sales, R. (2002) The deserving and the undeserving? Refugees, asylum seekers and welfare in Britain, *Critical Social Policy*, 22(3): 456–78.

Sidoti, C. (2002) Refugee Policy: is there a way out of this mess, In Human Rights and Equal Opportunity Commission (ed.), *Racial Respect Seminar*, Human Rights and Equal Opportunity Commssion, Canberra.

Steiner, N. (2000) *Arguing about asylum: the complexity of refugee debates in Europe*, St Martin's Press, New York.

Taran, P. (2000) Human rights of migrants: challenges of the new decade, *International Migration*, 38(6): 7–51.

UNHCR (1951) *Convention relating to the status of refugees*, UNHCR, Geneva.

UNHCR (1967) *Protocol relating to the status of refugees*, UNHCR, Geneva.

UNHCR (1999) *EXCOM Conclusions: no. 44*, UNHCR, Geneva.

Notes

1 References to the 1951 Refugee Convention throughout this volume are to the 1951 Convention Relating to the Status of Refugees done at Geneva on 28 July 1951 and the 1967 Protocol Relating to the Status of Refugees done at Geneva on 31 January 1967.

2 Global IDP Project (2002) *A Global Overview of Internal Displacement*, Norwegian Refugee Council, Geneva.

3 Universal Declaration of Human Rights, adopted and proclaimed by the United Nations General Assembly resolution 217A(III) on 10 December 1948.

4 This is complemented by Article 26, which states that 'All persons are equal before the law and are entitled without any discrimination to the equal protection of the law.'

2

Forced Migration, Globalisation, and Public Health: Getting the Big Picture into Focus

Anthony B. Zwi and Fatima Alvarez-Castillo

Introduction: Linking forced migration, public health, and globalisation

Interacting political, economic, and environmental factors impel people to migrate. Those affected are people who are typically vulnerable to start with, and who then take, or are forced to take, the difficult decision to leave their homes and move in order to seek better opportunities of survival (Richmond 1994). Human mobility is an integral part of the biological and cultural evolution of human settlement. The spread of populations, cultural innovation, and developments in technology were made possible when people came into contact with others and when they settled in new territories. Forced population movements in earlier stages of human evolution resulted from conflict, the slave trade, death and disease, and natural calamities.

Forced migration has distinctive features. Using the framework on human agency developed by Giddens (1984), Richmond differentiated migration which is proactive (voluntary) from migration which is reactive (forced), while acknowledging the fuzzy border between these. Most migrations take place somewhere between these poles where people have either a relatively high degree of agency and those whose autonomy is extremely limited. In most cases, those migrating seek to use available information to make choices, which aim to minimise risks and maximise potential advantages (proactive migration). However, many forced migrants make decisions in a 'state of panic during a crisis that leaves few alternatives but escape from intolerable threats' (reactive migration). Proactive migrants are often considered to be 'economic migrants', ineligible for refugee status, and they typically fall outside the ambit of protection through the United Nations (UN) Refugee Convention. The majority of those classified as refugees are reactive migrants, forced to move or flee (Richmond 1994).

Trends in forced migration

Forced migration is a general term used to describe involuntary movement by groups of people. Such populations are often responding to threats or experience of violence. The result is people moving across borders as refugees or within countries as internally displaced people. Some features of their numbers, trends, and patterns are described below.

The First and Second World Wars resulted in massive transfers of populations between states, especially within Europe. After decolonisation in Africa, prolonged periods of displacement resulted from repressive regimes, conflict, and external destabilisation campaigns and interventions (Schmeidl 2001). Chronic ongoing conflict has continued to this day in many decolonised countries, including Angola, Burundi, Chad, Rwanda, Sudan, Uganda, and Zaïre/Congo. In Asia massive flows of forced migrants accompanied the partition of India and formation of Pakistan in 1947. Large outflows also occurred as a result of the suppression of Tibetan autonomy (1956–59), the Chinese Cultural Revolution, the Indo-Chinese conflict affecting Vietnam, Laos, and Cambodia, and the internal conflict with minority communities in Burma/Myanmar. In addition, separatist struggles in Sri Lanka, the southern Philippines, and Indonesia have all led to extensive forced migration. In Latin America, massive populations of forced migrants accompanied the struggles for social transformation in some of the poorest and most stratified nations in the region: Nicaragua, El Salvador, and Guatemala (Schmeidl 2001). In the Middle and Near East the main contributors to forced migration were the exoduses of Palestinians accompanying the formation of the state of Israel in 1948 and the Six Day War in 1967, and the Afghans, fleeing violence or repression. In the former Soviet Union and Eastern Bloc, major movements of population accompanied regime changes and periods of revolt in the years after World War II and then in the period after the end of the Cold War, during which major conflicts occurred in the former Yugoslavia, Georgia, Moldova, Tajikistan, Armenia, Uzbekistan, and Azerbaijan.

While the immediate end of World War II saw 'wholesale population shifts on a deliberate basis', with Germans expelled by Poland (9 million) and by Czechoslovakia (3 million) (Lyons 1999), the subsequent period saw the use of refugee flows as a political issue. The USA, for example, through its funding support for refugee programs, had on a number of occasions, exercised influence on UN policy regarding admission or rejection of refugees in consideration of ideological rivalry (Lee et al. 2002; Zwi et al. 2002). Refugees have often been hostages in global conflicts, used as political pawns, or as a political buffer (Mayotte 1987). While refugees from 'enemy states' were seen as politically attractive as they demonstrated the failure of opposing political systems and hence were admitted to the host country, the vast majority of forced migrants were not. In summary, refugees were, and often continue to be, used for security, foreign policy, and economic gain.

Refugee numbers have risen from 2.5 million in 1970, to 11 million in 1983, 18.2 million in 1992 and 23 million in 1997 (Reed et al. 1998). Added to these numbers is an increase in internally displaced people, of whom, in the decade following the end of the Cold War, there were an estimated 30 million (Reed et al. 1998), the vast majority fleeing conflict zones.

In the two decades prior to 1990, there were 74 countries from which refugees had fled and 35 countries with internally displaced populations. In the period 1990–1995 there were 70 countries with populations in exile, and 51 with internally displaced populations. Almost all countries that had internally displaced populations also produced refugees who fled over the country's borders (Schmeidl 2001). In broad terms, more countries produced refugees than internally displaced people, and most countries with internally displaced populations also produced refugees. Work on internal displacement often lags behind forced migration across borders, and forced migration has become more globalised, affecting more countries in the post-Cold War period than earlier in the twentieth century (Schmeidl 2001).

Analysis of the provisional United Nations High Commissioner for Refugees (UNHCR) population statistics for 2000 demonstrates a number of key features (UNHCR 2000). In 2000 there were estimated to be at least 12.1 million refugees, the majority being hosted in Asia (5.4 million; 44 per cent) or Africa (3.6 million refugees; 30 per cent). Just over half of these, around 6.9 million persons, benefit from UNHCR assistance programs, which, again, are overwhelmingly located in Asia and Africa.

Among the key events in 2000 were the return of some 350,000 refugees in Asia to their home country, and another 160,000 in Europe. In all, approximately 800,000 refugees returned to their home countries in 2000, about half as many as in 1999. Remarkably, only 40,000 refugees were resettled in third countries with UNHCR assistance, a tiny fragment of the 12.1 million refugees noted earlier (UNHCR 2000).

The world's largest group of refugees were, in 2000, Afghans, number-ing some 3.6 million people and nearly 30 per cent of the global refugee burden. Burundians formed the second largest refugee nationality (5 per cent), followed by refugees from Iraq (4 per cent). Palestinians, are listed in separate statistics but are a longstanding refugee community, having fled or been forced from their homes over fifty years ago.

The UNHCR reported on 14 December 2001 on global refugee trends from January–September 2001. According to this report, there was a 4 per cent decrease in the refugee population in the 87 asylum countries listed during the period covered by the report. The ten asylum countries that reported the largest decrease were mostly in Africa; the rest were in the former Yugoslavia and the Russian Federation. The ten asylum coun-tries that reported the largest increase were all in Africa, except Thailand, Iraq, and Costa Rica. In the period covered by the report, the UNHCR assisted the voluntary repatriation of 110,000 refugees, all in Africa, with the exception of East Timorese refugees from Indonesia. Based on these data, Africa appeared to be the continent in which significant headway was made by the UN agency.

A key point to note is the tremendous pressure on already severely stretched resources for the developing countries as well as for interna-tional assistance, particularly of the UNHCR. On a number of occasions in the past decade, sudden flare-ups of conflict in the former Yugoslavia, Kosovo, Congo, East Timor, and Afghanistan, have led to calls for massive international assistance and UNHCR support, intensifying pressure on already meagre resources and depleting those for other ongoing chronic unresolved crises in other parts of the world. Forced migration flows may be immense, as in Kosovo where 800,000 people were forced to flee within days, requiring high levels of support.

Mechanisms to promote accountability to affected communities are in their infancy, with refugees in most situations being seen by many policy makers as passive participants in events unfolding around them. The ebb and flow of refugees and other displaced people are indications of the acceleration and deceleration of global and local conflict. The refugee problem serves as a mirror on the kinds of war that are being waged in today's world. Non-combatants, women, and entire communities are vic-timised. 'The modes of warfare are increasingly focused on destabilization and terror, specifically to undermine community structures in opposing groups through massacres of civilians, destruction and looting of neigh-bours and systematic rape' (Zwi et al. 2002).

While there had been periods of relative deceleration in refugee flow between the end of World War II and the present, the trend is towards an overall increase rather than decrease. The volume of repatriation and resettlement is generally small, although following major geopolitical changes such as the end of the NATO strikes against Yugoslavia in Kosovo, or the overthrow of the Taliban in Afghanistan, huge numbers of refugees have returned from surrounding countries.

Globalisation has changed the pattern of forced migration

The Carnegie Commission on Preventing Deadly Conflict identified a range of factors that contribute to the occurrence of violent political conflict (Carnegie Commission on Preventing Deadly Conflict 1997). Many of these are exacerbated by current processes of globalisation, which highlights widening inequities in the presence of increased competition, widespread availability of weapons, and a declining or worsening capacity of states to manage the political challenges inherent in such unstable situations and, ultimately, to maintain control over the exercise of force (Zwi et al. 2002).

Globalisation can be considered to be a multifaceted process affecting economic, political, social, and cultural spheres of activity (Lee et al. 2002). Collinson defines globalisation as a 'set of processes that are global in scope, that transcend the territorial borders of states and which, as a consequence, profoundly affect the nature and functions of state governance in the world political economy' (Collinson 1999).

There are a number of potential links between globalisation and forced migration, in part operating through increased risk of conflict and violence. A key element is the changing nature of the state. Since the early 1980s macroeconomic policy advice and pressure sought to downscale the state, promoted through structural adjustment policies (SAPs), supported by the IMF, the World Bank, global capital, and many high-income governments. Globalisation has helped promote neoliberal perspectives and has ensured the hegemony of such discourse through the global mass media, global financial institutions, and the UN. A weakened state predisposes, in many cases, to increased risk of violence (Zwi et al. 2002), especially where its ability and commitment to reducing inequities is minimal.

Second, the World Bank continues to strongly advocate that state economic policies must be responsive to 'the parameters of a globalised world economy', amplifying the state's changing role from provider to facilitator and regulator (World Bank 1997) and further undermining its role as a redistributor of resources and services. Thirdly, it is increasingly apparent that 'the opportunities and rewards of globalisation [are] spread unequally and inequitably—concentrating power and wealth in a select group of people, nations and corporations, marginalizing the others' (United Nations Development Program 1999). Thus while globalisation has brought about integration on some levels, it has contributed to fragmentation on others, dividing communities, nations, and regions. Income and wealth gaps are much wider in the developing world than the developed. Given that inequalities, especially those based on ethnic, religious, or cultural affiliation, are a potentially important cause of conflict, trends towards greater inequity as a result of current forms of globalisation, in the presence of intense resource constraints, may be a potent driver of violent political conflict.

Duffield (1994) argues that complex political emergencies are deeply politicised conflicts 'characteristic of areas of protracted economic crisis and growing social vulnerability'. This resonates for refugee-producing conflicts such as those in Afghanistan, Angola, or Sudan. While state failure is a critical element, conflict reflects a situation in which 'violence has become an important adjunct of economic and political survival in landscapes increasingly lacking alternatives' (Duffield 1994a). Social tensions and conflicts ignite in the presence of extreme inequality, not only of income and wealth, but also in political participation, access to economic assets (such as land, human capital, and communal resources) and social services (education, housing, health, and employment).

Many current conflicts occur in situations where state revenues have declined, economic constraints are great, corruption and inefficiency rife, and paramilitary groups that pillage and plunder are present (Duffield 2001). Kaldor (1999) describes the net effect as a blurring between barbarity and civility, combatants and non-combatants, and between soldier, policeman, and criminal.

Globalisation also has other interfaces with current conflicts (Zwi et al. 2002). Global communication technologies facilitate the construction of new ethnic identities by drawing together local and diaspora communities, allowing the rapid exchange of ideas, some hostile, which may foment violence and include the transfer of funds and resources that contribute to conflict. Phobic nationalism may be fostered by loss of control over foreign investment inflows and outflows, hostility to immigration, fears of unemployment, resentment of international institutions, fears of terrorism and subversion, hostility to global media, and the attractions of secession (Halliday 1997). Violent political conflict thus reflects a range of these influences and cannot be oversimplified as ethnic conflict, decontextualised from the reality of politics and economics (Allen & Seaton 1999).

The burden of forced migrants falls on developing countries not the wealthy North

While globalisation has had an impact upon the sovereignty of states, especially poor countries, there are many barriers to international agencies like the UNHCR deciding on requests for asylum. The primacy of states remains a strong principle in international law. It is the accepted rule of international law that any question as to whether a person possesses the nationality of a particular state should be determined in accordance with the laws of that state (Coquia & Sanitago 1998). Thus the UNHCR has to get the agreement of states on the refugee status of forced migrants. This has caused a substantial backlog in the number of refugees waiting for acceptance in host countries. Latter day forms of internal violence have tested the notion of sovereignty and its limits as the international community experiments with different forms of intervention response.

Although wealthy industrialised countries often complain of the burden of absorbing refugee populations, they do much less than poorer developing countries. The main refugee hosting countries are developing countries (UNHCR 2000). Pakistan in 2000 was host to over 2 million refugees, Iran 1.87 million, and Tanzania nearly 681,000. Of the industrialised countries, Germany and the United States were the two countries hosting the largest number of refugees, having absorbed in the decade prior to the year 2000, 906,000 and 507,300 refugees respectively. Of all refugees absorbed into other countries by 2000, little more than 20 per cent were in the highly industrialised countries, with poor countries such as Pakistan and Iran hosting nearly as many refugees in their own countries as in all the developed countries combined (UNHCR 2000).

Governments of wealthy countries discriminate against refugees who are considered to be a potential burden in terms of social security and health needs, whereas they have positive incentives for new migrants with skills and money to invest. It is to some extent ironic that wealthy countries do least for the poorest and most vulnerable of the world's population, while poor countries, such as Pakistan, Tajikistan, and Tanzania, are requested by the UN to open their borders to Afghan and central African refugees respectively, despite their indefinite length of stay.

It is important to note that there are also considerable inequities in how international humanitarian resources are made available to affected people. Funds for humanitarian crises in Kosovo were many orders of magnitude greater than those available in West Africa or Congo.

Internally displaced people are at even greater risk than refugees

The great majority of forced migrants are poor, in danger due to war, ethnic violence, political repression, widespread criminality, natural disasters, and in some cases, development activities. They are invariably people whose governments cannot provide protection or whose governments are the source of danger. Kofi Annan, the Secretary-General of the United Nations highlights their particular plight '…states are sometimes the principal perpetrator of violence against the very citizens that humanitarian law requires them to protect. Second, non-state combatants, particularly in collapsed states, are often ignorant or contemptuous of humanitarian law. Third, international conventions do not adequately address the specific needs of vulnerable groups, such as internally displaced persons, or women and children in complex emergencies' (Annan 2000).

Francis Deng, the Representative of the UN Secretary-General on internally displaced persons argues that 'What should be emphasized about internal displacement is that in most instances, the affected countries suffer from an acute crisis of national identity. This creates vacuums of responsibility for the displaced population and other victims of conflict situations. Instead of the government seeing the victims as citizens who should be protected and assisted, they are often seen as part of the enemy, and are therefore deprived of shelter, basic food, medicine—virtually all necessities for a reasonably decent living. In essence, these are a people dispossessed, abandoned by their own governments' (Deng 2000).

Those displaced within countries have less access to resources and support from the international community, and may be at ongoing risk from violence perpetrated by the state and other local actors (Collinson 1999; Hampton 1998). Moreover, established agencies such as the UNHCR are mandated to deal with refugees and not specifically with those internally displaced.

Not all those who need to escape danger can do so. Personal circumstances can prevent flight. Money is needed to travel, and may be used to bribe border guards or other officials. Contacts and prior knowledge are needed to identify the least dangerous escape routes. Women, the elderly, the infirm, disabled and very young may be left either to maintain a presence in the household, because they may not be deemed initially worth the investment required to get out, or because they may be considered a potential impediment to the speed of migration. Geographical factors can facilitate escape in some areas (e.g. shared land borders) but impede it in others (e.g. islands that necessitate crossing large bodies of water to get to safety). Boat people, those stored in container vehicles or railroads, may take considerable risks with death, a not uncommon adverse effect, in their efforts to reach safety and a more secure future.

Those who make it as refugees, who get over borders or are offered opportunities to seek asylum in third countries are, in many ways, much luckier than those internally displaced and still at risk from forces in their own country.

Female forced migrants are at particular risk

While minority communities, older people, and the infirm suffer increased risks, women in all these groups suffer an additional burden, whether as refugees, internally displaced people, or asylum seekers. These risks arise for a number of reasons: prevailing culture that justifies gender discrimination in societies in both North and South, resulting in various forms of abuse against women; gender inequity that deprives women of resources (e.g. food or health services) and the protection of the state; cultural structures which place women in positions subservient to the needs of men (use of women refugees to attend to the personal needs such as cooking, laundry, and sex for military or rebel officers), and the targeting of women for violent abuses such as rape in wartime. A cumulative effect of these circumstances is increased vulnerability of women to violence and abuse by both 'protective' and opposing forces.

Already victims of discrimination in the absence of war, women and girls are additionally exposed to sexual violence in many conflicts. The growing reality of total war in which the scope of war has widened so much that the civilian population is totally caught up in the fighting, has led to an increase in female-headed households as a result of the conscription of men, their detention, displacement or death (Benson 1994; Lindsey 2001). When women return home, they are highly vulnerable to sexual abuse by bandits, male refugees, and even those charged with protecting them (Kumar 1997).

While women may exhibit heightened resilience, they are also more vulnerable in some settings and circumstances. It may well be that those women who are most vulnerable because they are isolated, come from marginalised groups, and have fewer social networks, are at greatly increased risk. Women who have better systems of support may be in a better position to show agency, to seize control of situations, and demonstrate their inherent resilience. The experiences of women as refugees are further expanded in chapters six and seven.

Forced migration, public health, and accountability

Pre-existing health problems may be exacerbated during periods of forced migration (see Toole p. 35). These threats to health apply in the acute phase of displacement (Toole et al. 2001) but may continue in situations of chronic conflict, longstanding displacement, and even when they return home, if they ever do. Prior health status and access to food, shelter, water and sanitation, and health services, as well as the level of resource availability, all affect health prior to and as a result of conflict.

Forced migration places those forced to move at increased risk of ill health. In the absence of adequate forms of support to health systems responsible for providing care, the risks of ill-health may spread beyond the forced migrants to other populations, such as the host populations that shelter and support them. On the other hand, there are increasingly well-established methods for controlling communicable diseases among displaced populations, and if applied effectively and resourced appropriately, the risks to affected populations and their hosts may be substantially reduced. One problem is that available knowledge of best practice is often not applied, either because the information is not accessed when needed, or because there are impediments to its implementation.

Promoting policy accountability is on some agendas: questions are rightly asked of governments, United Nations agencies, transnational corporations, and civil society organisations, to explain their objectives, policies, strategies, and activities. Those providing funds, including the general public through taxation and charitable donations, want to see benefits from the resources provided. While valuable, this pushes agencies into providing services that can be counted, costed, and seen; whereas some necessary humanitarian actions are not immediately amenable to such analyses.

The UNHCR, as the pre-eminent body dealing with refugees, has been subjected to critique in relation to its role in protecting and serving internally displaced people, dealing with long-term chronic refugee situations, interacting with the private sector in providing services for displaced people, and contributing to longer-term development and post-conflict stability.

Non-governmental organisations (NGOs) are also under pressure to perform, to do and be seen to be doing, and to be seen to be doing well.

There are few incentives to reveal weaknesses or problems, even though failing to do so will perpetuate them. NGOs are not generally funded to reflect, analyse, and learn. There is emerging interest in placing experience on the table: the Sphere Project brought together humanitarian NGO networks to develop minimum standards for response to disasters (the Sphere Project 2000), the Humanitarian Accountability Project seeks to ensure that the voices of potential beneficiaries in emergencies are heard, and the Active Learning Network on Accountability and Performance (ALNAP) seeks to document and evaluate responses and improve performance and lesson-learning by humanitarian agencies.

Stoking fears: implications to public health

Public health has been defined as 'the art and science of preventing disease, promoting health, and prolonging life through organised efforts of society' (Committee of Inquiry into the Future Development of the Public Health Function 1988). According to Beaglehole and Bonita (1997) the essential elements of modern public health theory and practice are its emphasis on collective responsibility for health and the prime role of the state in protecting and promoting the public's health; a focus on whole populations; an emphasis on prevention; a concern for the underlying socio-economic determinants of health and disease; a multi-disciplinary basis that incorporates quantitative and qualitative methods as appropriate; and partnership with the population served (Beaglehole & Bonita 1997). Peace and security are widely recognised as essential elements for the broader promotion of health and the delivery of effective health care.

The protection of public health is not infrequently identified as one of the rationales for keeping refugees, asylum seekers, and other forced migrants out. The Refugee Council of Australia drew attention in 2000 to allegations of refugees and boat people as 'carriers of disease' (Refugee Council of Australia 2000).

In the wake of September 11, but even in the years preceding it, more and more issues have been defined as 'security issues'. The security concerns are typically presented in terms of national security, focusing attention on the need to protect the interests of Western democratic states and their economic underpinnings. The paper by Moodie and Taylor (2000) suggests that there is need to consider much more precisely the interface between public health and security, arguing that 'it is clear that policymakers and analysts concerned with national security must focus on the intersections of health and international security', although they recognise that an understanding of these interactions is at an early stage. They quote Lute in a report to the Carnegie Commission on Preventing Deadly Conflict as describing complex emergencies as resulting from the entanglement of four scourges: war, disease, hunger, and displacement, issues that are at the core of this chapter.

In considering the public health response, we need to be careful that public health does not simply service those concerned with national security. There is a real risk of this occurring given that the security 'industry' has found cause in raising fears of infection and disease spreading from conflict-affected areas to the rest of the globe. Furthermore, the public health community has grabbed the new interest in emerging and re-emerging infections as a means of mobilising both public interest and funds. Indirectly this has implicitly placed public health as a junior party to bigger concerns with security. This also implies that those affected by disease and infection, such as some forced migrants, are less important in their own right than the needs of wealthy industrialised countries that seek to control the emergence and resurgence of infectious diseases.

Keeping people out of the nation state, as attempted by Australia in its so-called Pacific Plan, whereby refugees and asylum seekers have their claims processed in small Pacific island states without entering Australian territory is one manifestation of this. A counter-productive effect of this is that in at least one such processing centre detained refugees and asylum seekers were at more risk of malaria than at any time previously.

There is no doubt that refugees and asylum seekers are an emotive issue everywhere: whether in Britain, France, South Africa, Pakistan, Thailand, or Australia. Virtually everybody has an opinion, whether well informed or otherwise. Populist political parties routinely drum up fears around migrants, refugees, and asylum seekers in an effort to stoke up support for narrowly constructed visions of national interest, which is often xenophobic and vicious in both content and form. Fortress Europe is a common refrain as many states seek to collectively keep out a perceived swarm of people from the former Soviet Union, North Africa and the Indian and Chinese subcontinents (Steiner 2000).

The Australian federal elections of 2001 were, at least in part, won by the sitting Liberal Party, on the back of victim-blaming data and images regarding boat people, refugees, and asylum seekers. Those seeking protection and safety were cast as jumping the queue, throwing their children into the sea, bringing disease into the country, and after September 11, of being potential terrorists. As remarked by Zolberg (2001), international migration has 'ascended to the status of a security issue, imperatively requiring attention in the highest places'. However, the reflex responses which many forced migration issues elicit are often counterproductive and excessively harsh, as identified by Sen (cited by Zolberg) 'the emergency mentality based on false beliefs in imminent cataclysms leads to breathless responses that are deeply counterproductive' (Zolberg 2001). Draconian measures taken to protect sovereignty and human flows across international borders are often at the expense of seemingly more banal humanitarian obligations.

Migrants' contexts and resilience: a more complete picture

In the interest of promoting the health of the whole population, particularly including the vulnerable, public health practitioners have a responsibility to transcend the political debates and ensure that information on which policy is based is more complete. There is an overwhelming literature and media coverage of the negative aspects of forced migration and of the rising demand being placed on wealthy states. Industrialised countries hear about stories of victimhood. The prevailing impression that refugees are a social burden or threats to the security or ecology of host countries has been critiqued earlier in this chapter. In spite of the lack of evidence, this has been used to justify policies that are hostile to applicants for refugee status or immigration (Richmond 1994).

Evidence of resilience, of survival despite adversity, and of contributions being made by refugees, asylum seekers, and other forced migrants to their new countries is not adequately documented and made part of mainstream discourse. Migrants to Australia and Canada, for example, had, on average, higher occupational status and earnings than native-born Canadians or Australians (Beaujot et al. 1988; Birrell & Birrell 1987). The overall contributions of immigrants to Canadian society were recognised by former Canadian Prime Minister Pierre Trudeau who advanced a policy of multiculturalism towards an ethnically plural Canadian society (Richmond 1994). Despite resistance from many quarters, the debates that followed contributed to greater public knowledge about the benefits to Canadian society from immigrant communities, including enrichment of Canada's cultures, the arts as well as to education and scientific enterprises.

In her case study of experiences of forced migrants, Mayotte (1987) documented the relationship of mutual help that developed between Eritrean refugees in Sudan and local, rural communities in the country. Exchange of knowledge about folk medicine, small scale trading and intermarriages were among the activities that brought the two populations together. A sense of community began to develop between these groups, which helped both refugees and the local community to collectively respond to certain critical needs.

While traditional explanations suggest that communities undergoing severe stress of culture loss and resettlement tend to withdraw and embrace previous traditions (Scudder 1993), others (Krulfeld & Bridling 1993) suggest that the refugee situation can be an opportunity for positive change, including the construction of new gender roles and relationships. There is clearly a need to look at variations in context and experience and not to homogenise or dehumanise refugees.

Forced migrants are not a homogeneous group, even when fleeing the same conflict zone or economic hardships. Populations are differentiated by their class, religion, socio-economic status, political affiliation, and even state of health. Indigenous communities, the poor, women, elderly people, and those disabled may be additionally disadvantaged in many settings. Vulnerability differs among groups that also have differential exposure to risk, ability to cope, and to seize agency and control. The capacity to seek asylum in foreign lands has a class dimension with those most vulnerable often having to take the most extreme risks such as boarding unsafe boats or cashing in their remaining assets to pay people traffickers to transport them to another land.

A crucial advantage of highlighting positive migrant responses is the potential for reconstruction in the public mind as well as in public health of a prevailing paradigm, a core assumption of which is that migrants are a threat and a burden. This can get translated into improved policy response and provision of services, particularly when those most affected are directly involved. By grounding the narratives of communities of forced migrants in relevant socio-cultural and historical contexts, we may encourage democratic pluralism, which is an antidote to the cultural hegemonisation and homogenisation that otherwise arguably characterises contemporary globalisation.

The experiences and insights of affected communities must be brought to the core of policy making and program planning. Forced migrants must have a role in determining what services are provided and how. In the absence of this, resources may be misdirected, culturally inappropriate, not geared to the real needs of the particular populations concerned, and inequitably and insensitively distributed. Agency resides with those most affected: their ability to influence their environment needs support. Displaced people have pride and dignity, coping strategies, ideas, and resilience: these need to be understood and bolstered.

It is in its interests that the international community acts, and it is to assist them that services are provided. Are we doing enough to ensure that their voices are not only recorded, but are listened to? Have we grappled enough with the techniques of ensuring that the real-life experiences of people on the ground contribute to the development of more people-centred and humane emergency and development policies?

There are, of course, significant challenges in beginning to ensure that the stories of forced migrants are heard. People who have been excluded from the domain of public discourse, and who may be suffering from distress, loss, and exile, cannot easily speak about their lives. Noble intentions by researchers or aid givers do not necessarily create a resolve by affected people to participate in public or to explain their lives, experiences, past or future. It is important to recognise that the social value of research is not only in knowledge production but in helping people heal their various wounds, build their agency and locus of control. Emerging approaches and techniques evolved by feminist researchers who are concerned with making research an enabling experience for women, offer possibilities in this regard (Fonow and Cook, 1991; Harding, 1991; Oakley, 1992).

Promote a more humane globalisation

Globalisation provides a powerful backdrop to forced migration. It exemplifies the interconnectedness of people, places, and ideas over time and space. Globalisation challenges our responses to forced migration—questioning processes of governance and accountability of all actors in a world in which the role of the nation-state and multilateral organisations is contested—while civil society organisations and the private sector are touted as a major part of the solution. New technologies provide important mechanisms for enhancing debate, promoting accountability, learning lessons and listening to the voices and experiences of affected people.

Globalisation is ongoing. Reshaping it is crucial. The form which globalisation has taken to date leaves much to be desired. It has been driven primarily by the interests of the wealthier states, and by elites within poorer states. While it draws states closer together and lowers barriers across the globe, it also fragments, by sloughing off those territories and peoples who are less able, for historical and other reasons, to compete at the level and in the forums required. Globalisation may be disempowering for many, at times contributing to increasing inequities both within and between states.

Promoting a more humane globalisation is key to stemming the tide of forced migrants in the future. The globalisation of the media has both positive and negative features (see chapter fourteen). One positive side is the potential to increase more widespread awareness of conflicts and forced migration, and of the human misery they produce. The risks include oversimplifying the complexity of these situations. Little attention is devoted to understanding the underlying structural causes of the conflicts which produce forced migrants, nor of related contributors such as the global arms trade, widening social inequalities, and in some cases the activities of transnational corporations.

The availability of new technologies such as the Internet, offers opportunities to broaden awareness of and understanding around conflicts and their causes. Civil society groups, local communities, and scholars around the world continue to raise unrecognised issues that could be shared more widely in the public domain.

Information sharing may also increase transparency and accountability of the 'humanitarian industry'. Demand for evidence of the effectiveness and efficiency of humanitarian interventions should contribute to improvements in practice. As 'good practice' needs to be context-sensitive, drawing insights from a variety of settings and clarifying their specificities will be essential (Fustukian & Zwi 2001). Debates on key concerns, such as effective mechanisms for working with the military in delivering humanitarian assistance, or the role of a humanitarian ombudsman to ensure that neglected communities can articulate their concerns, deserve attention. Mechanisms for bolstering the resilience of individuals, communities and systems to the ill-effects of violent political conflict need to be developed and promoted, as is better understanding of the determinants and contributors to violent political conflict. Failure to identify and address root causes prior to, and in the aftermath of, conflict is likely to set up a new cycle of violence and retribution.

Current forms of globalisation appear to be inherently conflict-producing rather than conflict-diminishing. The United Nations Development Programme (UNDP) has called for a more humane globalisation that includes improving systems of global governance, reversing the most extreme forms of marginalisation, and seeking more actively to eradicate widespread poverty (United Nations Development Programme 1999). These and related interventions are necessary if the most negative effects of globalisation, many of which are associated with collective violence between states, but more particularly within states, are to be reduced. More action needs to be taken earlier and more effectively if such crises are to be avoided. 'Public health practitioners have a responsibility to draw attention to the importance of the linkage between human rights and public health and to develop methods of assessing the impact on human rights of health policies and programmes and health reforms' (Gostin & Mann 1994).

The humanitarian response can be improved through better information and structures that help identify countries and regions at risk of collective violence, encourage earlier intervention where appropriate, ensure ethical practices by the humanitarian industry, and hold to account those guilty of crimes against humanity. The globalising mass media has made the work of organisations like UNICEF, ICRC, and MSF more familiar to us all. While there are enhanced opportunities for hearing the voices of those most marginalised and adversely affected by global instability and conflict, it remains unclear whether we will make the effort to hear, or even more importantly, listen to these voices. The public health community has a major task to play in ensuring that we do.

At a broad international or even supra-national level, other challenges remain. A key issue is to identify the means to promote collective identities in pluralistic terms as a contribution to discouraging ethnic conflict (Robertson 1990). Among the mechanisms that have opened out in order to promote a more inclusive approach are the establishment and enrichment of more horizontal structures such as global networks and the establishment of international communities as active players in the field. Globalisation has opened the door to developing not only economic and political transfers and frameworks, but also global civil society working on such matters as human rights and humanitarian issues. Deacon (1999) has referred to the 'globalization of social policy and the socialization of global politics'. Evidence is certainly present of the massive growth in such organisations, reflecting the new technologies that facilitate global networking and the increasingly important role of such bodies in influencing media and public opinion, and through them, political decision making. International communities of this sort find common ground and purpose, operate as collectivities, building multi-vocal global platforms, and calling for changes in who holds power and how it is exercised.

Enhanced technologies may also stimulate an increase in mechanisms for demanding and monitoring how power is used, thus enhancing accountability and transparency. Both wealthy and poorer countries may be subject to such influences, given the role of international public opinion and multilateral aid in many settings.

The funding system for the United Nations requires change if more independent voices are to be heard and policy is to be influenced by evidence and not just the power of the players involved. Such an engagement also begins to transform how civil society operates, moving from nation-oriented to humanity-grounded and allowing the creation of spaces in which global platforms for advocacy emerge.

Conclusions

This chapter has set out to argue that practitioners working with forced migrants, refugees and asylum seekers would benefit from a broader appreciation of the 'big issues' affecting forced migrants. Appreciating why forced migrants flee, and their experiences, will allow practitioners to offer responsive services. We suggest also that public health practitioners can play a part in transforming the views that the lay public has about refugees. In order to do so, highlighting the moral and humanitarian commitment to supporting those forced to flee, and trumpeting the resilience and survival of those facing significant adversity, is critical. As practitioners we can play some part in making more visible the experiences of forced migrants and the communities they live in; and we can draw attention to the role of such forced migrants in widening the diversity and linkages between the global North and South.

We suggest that globalisation has been a major contributor to increasing levels of forced migration, in part for economic needs, but also in response to violent political change. We have suggested that public health practitioners should play some part in highlighting the inequities that result from current forms of globalisation, and that we should collectively play some part in identifying those which increase the gaps between the rich and poor, both within and between countries. Beaglehole and Bonita (1997) suggest that there is increasing scope for public health playing a more central role in human affairs: 'The economic pendulum will swing back towards a more collectivist approach as the ill-effects of the free market are recognised, especially by the huge marginalised segments of the world's population'.

The chapter has also sought to provide some comparative perspective in who is most at risk and the role of the countries that host refugees and asylum seekers. We draw particular attention to the fact that developing countries bear by far the greatest burden of caring for and supporting forced migrants. Only a tiny fraction of such people are ever resettled in wealthy countries of asylum. In fact, refugees themselves are better off than many other forced migrants, notably internally displaced people who do not cross international borders and may continue to be targeted and discriminated against by their own governments, which should be protecting them. Lastly, we argue that within populations of forced migrants, women are at greatest risk given levels of gender discrimination in most societies. Furthermore, the international protection mechanisms give only limited attention to the additional levels of vulnerability and risk faced by women in forced migration settings: they may be targeted by personnel supposedly 'on their side', by men in the services that are meant to be assisting and protecting them, and by their opponents.

We suggest that attention to context will improve both the quality and insight which practitioners bring to their work. This chapter highlights a set of issues we would do well to understand better—it does not provide answers—but suggests at least a number of avenues worth exploring. Ignoring context desensitises our responses; appreciating context allows our policies and interventions to be more fine-tuned to real needs and solutions to have a greater chance of success. Without an understanding and response to context, forced migrants will continue to flee and to flow and receiving nations will continue to fear.

Recommended readings

Global IDP Project (2002) *Internally Displaced People: A Global Survey*, Earthscan Publications, London.
UNHCR (2002) *Global Report 2001*, UNHCR Geneva.
Vincent, M. & Sorenson, B.R. (2002) *Caught Between Borders: Response Strategies of the Internally Displaced*, Pluto Press in association with NRC, London.
Zwi, A., Fustukian, S. & Sethi, D. (2002) Globalisation, conflict and the humanitarian response, In Buse, K., Fustukian, S. & Lee, K. (eds) *Health Policy in a globalising world*, Cambridge University Press, Cambridge, pp. 229–50.

References

Allen, T. & Seaton, J. (eds) (1999) *The media of conflict: war reporting and representations of ethnic violence*, Zed Books, London.
Annan, K. (2000) *We the people: the role of the United Nations in the 21st Century*, Report of the UN Secretary-General to the Millennium Assembly, In United Nations Organisation, Geneva, http://www.un.org/millennium/sg.report/ch3.pdf.
Beaglehole, R. & Bonita, R. (1997) *Public Health at the Crossroads. Achievements and Prospects*, Cambridge University Press, Cambridge.
Beaujot, R., Basavarajappa, K. & Verna, R. (1988) *Income of immigrants in Canada*, Statistics Canada, Ottawa.
Benson, J. (1994) 'Reinterpreting Gender: Southeast Asian Refugees and American Society', In Camino, L. & Krulfeld, R. (eds) *Reconstructing Lives, Recapturing Meanings: refugee identity, gender and cultural change*, Gordon and Breach, Amsterdam.
Birrell, R. & Birrell, T. (1987) *An issue of people: population and Australian society* (2nd edn), Longman Cheshire, Melbourne.

Carnegie Commission on Preventing Deadly Conflict (1997) *Preventing Deadly Conflict: Final Report*, Carnegie Corporation of New York, New York.

Collinson, S. (1999), 'Globalisation and the dynamics of international migration: implications for the refugee regime', In *New Issues in Refugee Research: Working Paper no 1*, Centre for Documentation and Research, UNHCR, Geneva, http://www.unhcr.ch/refworld/pubs/pubon.htm.

Committee of Inquiry into the Future Development of the Public Health Function (1988) Public Health in England, HMSO, cmd 289, London.

Coquia, J. & Sanitago, M. (1998) *International Law*, Central Professional Books, Quezon City, Philippines.

Deacon, B. (1999) 'Social policy in global context', In Hurrell, A. & Woods, N. (eds) *Inequality, globalization and world politics*, Oxford University Press, Oxford, pp. 211–47.

Deng, F. (2000) 'Conclusion: The cause of justice behind civil wars', In Amadiume, I. & An-Na'im, A. (eds) *The politics of memory. Truth, healing and social justice*, Zed Books, London, pp. 184–200.

Duffield, M. (1994a) 'Complex emergencies and the crisis of developmentalism', *IDS Bulletin*, 25(4): 37–45.

Duffield, M. (1994b) 'The political economy of internal war: asset transfer, complex emergencies and international aid', In Macrae, J. & Zwi, A. (eds) *War and hunger. Rethinking international responses to complex emergencies*, Zed Books, London, pp. 50–69.

Duffield, M. (2001) *Global Governance and the New Wars. The merging of development and security*, Zed Books, London.

Fustukian, S. & Zwi, A. (2001) *Balancing imbalances: facilitating community perspectives in times of adversity. Caring for those in crisis: integrating anthropology and public health in complex humanitarian emergencies*, National Association for the Practice of Anthropology, NAPA Bulletin, 21: 17–35.

Giddens, A. (1984) *The Constitution of Society*, Polity Press, Cambridge.

Gostin, L. & Mann, J. (1994) 'Towards the development of a human rights impact assessment for the formulation and evaluation of health policies', *Health and Human Rights*, 1: 6–23.

Halliday, F. (1997) 'Nationalism', In eds, Baylis, J. & Smith, S. (eds) *The globalization of world politics: an introduction to international relations*, Oxford University Press, Oxford.

Hampton, J. (1998) *Internally displaced people: a global survey*, Earthscan, London.

Kaldor, M. (1999) *New and old wars: organized violence in a global era*, Polity Press, Cambridge.

Krulfeld, R. & Bridling, L. (1993) 'New paradigms of methods and theory in culture change from refugee studies and related issues of power and empowerment', In Hopkins, M.C. & Donnelly, N. (eds), *Selected papers on refugee issues*, American Anthropology Association, Washington DC, pp. 29–41.

Kumar, K. (1997) *Rebuilding Societies After Civil War: Critical Roles for International Assistance*, Lynn Reiner, Colorado.

Lindsey, C. (2001) *Women Facing War*, ICRC Study on the Impact of Armed Conflict on Women, International Committee of the Red Cross, Geneva.

Lyons, M. (1999) *World War II: A Short History*, Prentice Hall, New Jersey.

Mayotte, J. (1987) *Disposable people: the plight of refugees*, Orbis Books, New York.

Moodie, M. & Taylor, W. (2000) *Contagion and conflict. Health as a global security challenge*, Chemical and Biological Arms Control Institute and CSIS International Security Program.

Reed, H., Haaga, J. & Keely, C. (eds) (1998) *The demography of forced migration*, Summary of a workshop, National Academy Press, Washington DC.

Refugee Council of Australia (2000), *Discussion Paper on the Response to the 1999–2000 Boat Arrivals*, available at: http://www.refugeecouncil.org.au/position01032000.htm.

Richmond, A. (1994) *Global Apartheid: Refugees, Racism and the New World Order*, Oxford University Press, Oxford.

Robertson, R. (1990) 'Mapping the Global Condition: Globalization as the Central Concept', In Featherstone, M. (ed.), *Global culture, nationalism, globalization and modernity*, Sage, London.

Schmeidl, S. (2001) 'Conflict and forced migration: a quantitative review, 1964–1995', In Zolberg, A. & Benda, P. (eds) *Global migrants, global refugees. Problems and solutions*, Berghan Books, Oxford, pp. 62–94.

Scudder, T. (1993) 'The human ecology of big river projects: river basin development and settlement', *American Review of Anthropology*, 2: 45–61.

Steiner, N. (2000) *Arguing about asylum: the complexity of refugee debates in Europe*, St Martin's Press, New York.

Sphere Project, The (2000) *Humanitarian Charter and Minimum Standards in Disaster Response*, The Sphere Project, Geneva.

Toole, M.J., Waldman, R.J. & Zwi, A. (2001) 'Complex Humanitarian Emergencies', In Merson, M., Black, R. & Mills, A. (eds), *Textbook of International Public Health. Diseases Programs, Systems and Policies*, Aspen Publications, Gaithersburg, Maryland, pp. 439–513.

UNHCR (2000) *Global refugee trends*, analysis of the 2000 provisional UNHCR statistics, UNHCR, Geneva.

United Nations Development Programme (1999), Human Development Report 1999, In World Bank (1997), *The state in a changing world*, Oxford University Press, Oxford.

Zolberg, A. (2001) 'Introduction: beyond the crisis', In Zolberg, A. & Benda, P. (eds), *Global migrants, global refugees. Problems and solutions*, Berghahn Books, New York, pp. 1–16.

Zwi, A., Fustukian, S. & Sethi, D. (2002) 'Globalisation, conflict and the humanitarian response', In Buse, K., Fustukian, S. & Lee, K. (eds), *Health Policy in a globalising world*, Cambridge University Press, Cambridge, pp. 229–50.

3

The Health of Refugees: an International Public Health Problem

Mike Toole

Introduction

During the past fifty years, approximately 600,000 refugees and displaced persons from Asia, Africa, Latin America, and Europe have been resettled in Australia (Australian Department of Immigration and Multicultural and Indigenous Affairs 2001). Very few of these people sought asylum directly in Australia; the vast majority were selected for resettlement in countries of first asylum. While almost 50 per cent of the refugees resettled in Australia during the past decade have come from Eastern Europe, many others have spent long periods in low-income countries of first asylum, such as Iran, Pakistan, Kenya, Ethiopia, Thailand, Guinea, and Honduras. They have fled armed conflicts and long periods of deprivation in their homelands to be temporarily housed in large sprawling camps that have often lacked the basic requirements for health and well-being. In this chapter, the magnitude of the international refugee problem is reviewed, the major health problems affecting refugees are examined, and the most important public health priorities in refugee assistance programs are summarised.

The number of dependent refugees under the protection and care of the United Nations High Commissioner for Refugees (UNHCR) steadily increased from approximately six million in thirty-eight countries in 1980 to almost 20 million in 1990. By 1998, the number declined to about 13.5 million due to a number of large repatriations of refugees to their homelands (United States Committee for Refugees 1998). Since 1998 the global number of refugees has risen again and remained greater than 14 million as a result of conflicts in Kosovo, East Timor, Sierra Leone, and Afghanistan (see figure 3.1). In addition, some three million

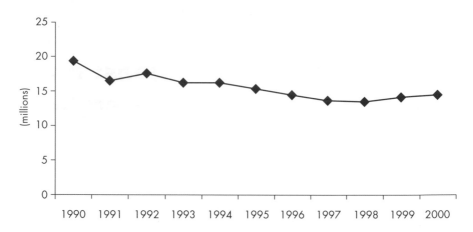

Figure 3.1 Estimated global number of refugees (millions) 1990–2000

Palestinian refugees, assisted by the UN Relief and Works Agency, are to be found on the West Bank, in Gaza and other parts of the Middle East.

Several of the world's largest-ever mass migrations took place in the last decade of the twentieth century. For example, in 1991, as many as one million Kurdish refugees fled Iraq for Iran or Turkey following the Gulf War. By early 1993 there were at least 1.5 million refugees or displaced persons within the republics of the former Yugoslavia. Between April and July 1994, an estimated two million Rwandan refugees fled into Tanzania, Eastern Zaïre, and Burundi provoking the most serious refugee crisis in twenty years. Between March and June 1999, approximately 780,000 ethnic Albanians fled the Serbian province of Kosovo. This represented more than 50 per cent of the Albanian population of the province prior to the war. During the violence and destruction that followed the August 1999 referendum on independence in East Timor, between 300,000 and 400,000 people were displaced (almost 50 per cent of the population), of whom approximately 260,000 were forcibly moved into Indonesian-controlled West Timor.

Prior to 1990 most of the world's refugees had fled countries that ranked among the poorest in the world, such as Afghanistan, Cambodia, Mozambique, and Ethiopia. However, during the following decade, an increasing number of refugees originated in relatively more affluent countries, such as Kuwait, Iraq, the former Yugoslavia, Armenia, Georgia, Russia, and Azerbaijan. Nevertheless, the reasons for the flight of refugees generally remain the same: war, civil strife, and persecution. Hunger, while sometimes a primary cause of population movements is all too frequently only a contributing factor.

In addition to those persons who meet the international definition of refugees, millions of people have fled their homes for the same reasons as refugees but remain *internally displaced* in their countries of origin. It has not proven easy to ascertain the number and location of the world's internally displaced persons (IDP). This is due not only to definitional difficulties, but is also the result of several institutional, political, and operational obstacles. Despite these difficulties, there was a broad consensus that the global population of IDPs stood somewhere in the region of 20 million at the end of 2000. IDPs lack the protection afforded by the international conventions and protocols on refugees. Nevertheless, the Geneva Conventions and certain articles of the United Nations Charter afford some protection to IDPs. During the 1990s, the United Nations took some extraordinary measures to protect these populations in Southern Sudan, Northern Iraq, the republics of the former Yugoslavia, Somalia, and East Timor.

The World Bank estimates that between 90 and 100 million people around the world have been forcibly displaced over the past decade as a result of large-scale development initiatives such as dam construction, urban development, and transportation programs. An unknown number have also been uprooted by lower-profile forestry, mining, game park and land-use conversion projects. The scale of such displacement seems unlikely to diminish in the future, given the processes of economic development, urbanisation and population growth that are taking place in many low and middle-income countries (United States Committee for Refugees 2001).

Health consequences of displacement

The most common response to mass population movements is to establish camps or settlements; conditions in these camps have varied enormously. For example, camps for Rwandan refugees in eastern Zaïre in 1994 contained up to 300,000 persons; they were poorly planned and laid out, had inadequate sanitation, and poor access to clean water. It was difficult if not impossible to establish equitable distribution systems of food and shelter materials, and there was a high frequency of violence and other crimes. By contrast, smaller refugee camps in Burundi were more easily managed and suffered fewer health consequences related to environmental conditions.

In low-income countries, refugees and displaced populations have commonly experienced high rates of communicable diseases and malnutrition resulting in significant excess mortality. In general, the major

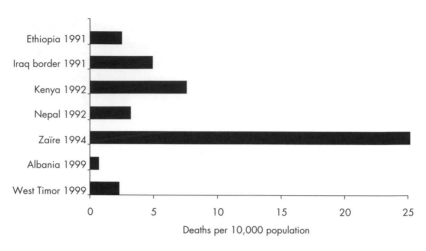

Figure 3.2 Mortality rates of selected refugee populations

health problems of refugees and internally displaced persons are similar in nature. However, the health status of the internally displaced may be worse because access to these populations by international relief agencies is often difficult and dangerous. Also, internally displaced persons may suffer more injuries because they are usually located closer to zones of conflict than are refugees; however, both refugees and internally displaced persons are often victims of landmines, particularly as they cross international borders.

Elevated mortality

The most severe health consequences of conflict and population displacement have occurred in the acute emergency phase, during the early stage of relief efforts, and have been characterised by extremely high mortality rates. Although the quality of the international community's disaster response efforts has steadily improved, death rates associated with forced migration have often remained high, as demonstrated by several emergencies during the 1990s (figure 3.2). For example, the exodus of almost one million Rwandan refugees into the Eastern Zaïre town of Goma in 1994 resulted in mortality rates that were more than 30 times the rates experienced prior to the conflict in Rwanda (Goma Epidemiology Group 1995). By contrast, the death rate among Kosovar refugees in Albania in 1999 was lower than the internationally recognised threshold of 'severe' (one death per 10,000 population per day) (Toole et al. 2001).

Trends in death rates over time have varied from place to place. In refugee populations, such as Cambodians in Eastern Thailand (1979) and Iraqis on the Turkish border (1991) where the international response has been prompt and effective, death rates have declined to baseline levels within one month. Among refugees in Somalia (1980) and Sudan (1985), death rates were still well above baseline rates six to nine months after the influx of refugees occurred (Toole & Waldman 1990). In the case of 170,000 Somali refugees in Ethiopia in 1988–89, death rates actually increased significantly six months after the influx. This increase was associated with elevated malnutrition prevalence, inadequate food rations, and high incidence rates of certain communicable diseases. Although initial death rates among Rwandan refugees in eastern Zaïre were extremely high, they declined dramatically within one to two months (Goma Epidemiology Group 1995).

Most deaths have occurred among children under 5 years of age; for example, 65 per cent of deaths among Kurdish refugees on the Turkish border occurred in the 17 per cent of the population less than 5 years of age (Yip & Sharp 1993). However, in some refugee situations, such as Goma during the first month after the refugee exodus, mortality rates were comparable in all age groups because the major cause of death was cholera, which is equally lethal at any age. In most reports from refugee camps, mortality rates have not been stratified by sex; however, the surveillance system for Burmese refugees in Bangladesh did estimate sex-specific death rates, demonstrating considerably higher death rates in females. Gendered analyses that take into account differences in the socio-cultural position of women have been rare in emergency settings.

The major reported causes of death among refugees and displaced populations in low-income countries have been diarrhoeal diseases, measles, acute respiratory infections, and malaria, exacerbated by high rates of malnutrition. These diseases consistently account for between 60 per cent and 95 per cent of all reported causes of death in these populations. In Eastern European conflicts, a high proportion of mortality among civilians has been caused by injuries associated with the violence. Nevertheless, there has also been increased mortality in these conflicts due to the collapse of the public health system. Chronic conditions, such as cardiovascular diseases, cancer, and renal conditions have been inadequately treated because the health system has focused on the management of war-related injuries.

Medical services in most parts of Bosnia and Herzegovina were overwhelmed by the demands of war casualties. The major hospital in Zenica reported that the proportion of all surgical cases associated with trauma

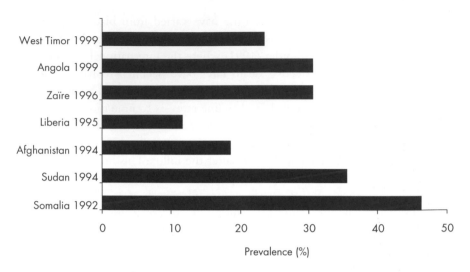

Figure 3.3 Prevalence of acute malnutrition, children less than 5 years, selected refugee and displaced population

steadily increased following the beginning of the war in April 1992, reaching 78 per cent in November of the same year (Toole et al. 1993). Preventive health services, including childhood immunisation and ante-natal care, ceased in many areas. The collapse of health services in Bosnia and Herzegovina had significant public health effects. For example, peri-natal mortality increased in Sarajevo from 16 deaths per 1000 live births in 1991 to 27 per 1000 during the first four months of 1993. The rate of premature births increased from 5.3 per cent to 12.9 per cent, the still-birth rate increased from 7.5 per 1000 to 12.3 per 1000, and the average birth weight decreased from 3700 grams to 3000 grams during the same period (Centers for Disease Control and Prevention 1993).

Malnutrition

Among refugees and IDPs, there are many factors that might lead to high rates of nutritional deficiency disorders, including prolonged food scarcity prior to and during displacement; delays in the provision of complete rations; problems with registration and estimation of the size of an affected population; and inequitable distribution systems. In general, the prevalence of acute malnutrition, or wasting, among children less than 5 years of age in low-income countries is between 5 per cent and 8 per cent. However, in refugee camps in these countries, the prevalence has often been between 20 per cent and 50 per cent accounting for the high fatality rate for common infectious diseases among children in these settings (figure 3.3). In contrast, acute malnutrition has been unusual among children in refugee and displaced populations in Eastern Europe where food scarcity has more commonly affected the elderly.

In some settings, refugee children who were adequately nourished upon arrival in camps have developed acute malnutrition due either to inadequate food rations or to severe epidemics of diarrhoeal disease. In the Hartisheik refugee camp in eastern Ethiopia, for example, the prevalence of acute malnutrition increased from less than 10 per cent to almost 25 per cent during a six-month period in late 1988 and early 1989 due to inadequate food rations (Toole & Bhatia 1992). In early 1991 the prevalence of acute malnutrition among Kurdish refugee children aged 12 to 23 months increased from less than 5 per cent to 13 per cent during a two-month period following a severe outbreak of diarrhoeal disease (Yip & Sharp 1993).

In Rwandan refugee camps in eastern Zaïre, the prevalence of acute malnutrition was between 18 per cent and 23 per cent following the severe cholera and dysentery epidemics during the first month after the influx (Goma Epidemiology Group 1995). Children with a history of dysentery within three days prior to the survey were three times more likely to be malnourished than those with no history of recent dysentery. Also, children in families headed by a woman were at significantly higher risk of malnutrition than those children in households headed by an adult male.

High incidence rates of several micronutrient deficiency diseases have been reported in many refugee camps, especially in Africa. Frequently, famine-affected and displaced populations have already experienced low levels of dietary vitamin A intake and, therefore, may have very low vitamin A reserves. Furthermore, the typical rations provided in large-scale relief operations lack vitamin A, putting these populations at high risk. In addition, those communicable diseases that are highly incident in refugee camps, such as measles and diarrhoea, are known to rapidly deplete vitamin A stores. Consequently, young refugee and displaced children are at high risk of developing vitamin A deficiency. In 1990 more than 18,000 cases of pellagra, caused by food rations deficient in niacin, were reported among Mozambican refugees in Malawi (Centers for Disease Control and Prevention 1991). Numerous outbreaks of scurvy (vitamin C deficiency) were documented in refugee camps in Somalia, Ethiopia, and Sudan between 1982 and 1991 (Desenclos et al. 1989). The prevalence of scurvy was highly associated with the period of residence in camps, a reflection of the time exposed to rations lacking in vitamin C.

Communicable diseases

The specific causes of mortality, and their age- and gender-distribution, do not differ from those that prevail in non-refugee populations. Accordingly, acute respiratory infections (ARI), diarrhoea, measles, and malaria have been most frequently cited as proximate causes. Substandard conditions found in camps do not change the diseases that account for most of the morbidity and mortality among refugees, but they do alter epidemiological patterns in two important ways. The incidence, or attack, rates of commonly occurring and potentially fatal diseases increase and the case-fatality rates (CFR) are higher than usual, probably because of increased malnutrition.

Measles

Measles has traditionally been among the most feared of communicable diseases in refugee camps. During the 1970s and 1980s, high incidence rates, particularly in populations with low levels of vaccination prior to displacement, high mortality rates, and unusually high CFRs, were typical of measles outbreaks among refugees. In an epidemic that occurred in the Wad Kowli refugee camp in Eastern Sudan in 1985, more than 3000 people out of a population of 80,000 died of this preventable condition during a six-month period. In well-vaccinated populations, such as Bosnian and Kosovar refugees in the Balkans, Kurds in Northern Iraq (1991), and Rwandans in Tanzania and Eastern Zaïre (1994), measles has been a less prominent public health problem.

Diarrhoea

Unlike measles, which can be easily prevented, diarrhoeal diseases remain one of the top three causes of mortality among refugees. In Somalia (1979–81), Ethiopia (1982), Sudan (1985), Malawi (1988), Northern Iraq (1991), and Goma (1994), diarrhoeal diseases were responsible for between 25 per cent and 85 per cent of all mortality. Although most often a condition of young children, cholera and dysentery, the major epidemic forms of diarrhoea, affect people of all ages. Of all disease conditions, diarrhoea is the most closely linked to poor sanitation, inadequate water quantity, contaminated water, and poor hygiene.

Cholera epidemics have occurred frequently in refugee and displaced populations. Although deaths due to non-cholera watery diarrhoea have been far more numerous, cholera, in addition to being able to cause death

rapidly from dehydration, incites fear and even panic in many populations. Its ability to affect other relief activities and to divert health personnel and supplies from other activities may even contribute to higher death
tolls due to other diseases. Outbreaks of cholera have occurred in all parts
of the world; large outbreaks were recorded among refugees in India
(1971), Thailand (1979), Sudan (1985), Somalia (1985), Ethiopia (1984),
Malawi (1988–91), Northern Iraq (1991), Goma (1994), and Rwanda
(1996).

Malaria

In endemic areas, including South-East Asia, the Indian subcontinent, and
most of Africa, malaria is consistently among the leading causes of morbidity and mortality. It was the leading cause of mortality among Cambodian
refugees in Thailand in 1978, Ethiopian refugees in Sudan in the mid 1980s,
and Mozambican refugees in Malawi in the 1980s. It has been well established that populations that are displaced to areas where malaria is more
highly endemic than their place of origin have higher incidence rates and
higher mortality. Following the collapse of health services and mass population displacement during and following the conflict in East Timor, the incidence of malaria increased significantly. In October 1999 approximately 30
per cent of all morbidity was attributed to malaria compared with 10 per
cent the previous year (World Health Organisation 1999).

Major risk factors for malaria in refugee situations include the lack of
adequate housing, poor location of camps (especially when they are
placed in marshy areas), overcrowding, proximity to livestock (which may
be the primary targets of mosquito vectors), and a general lack of compe-
tently trained health personnel. Although it has not been clearly documented in emergencies, the association of malaria with low birth weight
(especially in the offspring of first and second pregnancies) and with iron-
deficiency anaemia may cause increases in incidence and CFR from a
variety of causes, especially in children.

Other communicable diseases

Meningitis

Although not a consistent problem in refugee camps, the threat of Group
A meningococcal meningitis is a formidable one. Overcrowding, especially
during the drier seasons of the year, can be an important risk factor for this
disease, which is transmitted via the respiratory route. Large outbreaks have

occurred among refugees in Thailand (1980), Sudan (1989), Ethiopia (1993), Guinea (1993), and in Goma (1994). Outbreaks of meningitis tend to be protracted, lasting one to two months. Unless they are detected and controlled at an early stage, they can be directly responsible for high mortality; in addition, they can be resource-intensive and detract attention from other high-priority health programs.

Hepatitis E

Like meningitis, outbreaks of hepatitis E have not been frequent occurrences in refugee camps but have had major consequences when they occurred, especially among women. An enterically transmitted disease, usually linked to contaminated drinking water, hepatitis E is associated with a particularly high CFR in pregnant women. Clinical attack rates appear to be higher in adults, with children relatively spared. Large outbreaks have occurred in Somalia (1985), Ethiopia (1989), and among Somali refugees in Liboi Camp, Kenya (1991). In the latter outbreak, the overall case-fatality rate was 3.7 per cent but among pregnant women it was 14 per cent.

Tuberculosis

Tuberculosis (TB) is one of the most important communicable diseases to control in the post-emergency phase. Its re-emergence as a public health problem in many parts of the world is characterised by its close association with immune deficiency disorders, especially HIV/AIDS, and with the identification of multiple drug-resistant strains. TB can be quite common in some post-emergency situations. It is highly prevalent during the emergency as well, but because of the difficulties in developing programs to control its transmission, to diagnose and to reliably treat for adequate periods, other more acute conditions are appropriately accorded priority.

Sexually transmitted infections

HIV/AIDS and other STIs are major problems among persons displaced from areas where there is a high prevalence of these conditions. During the initial emergency phase, efforts to control HIV should focus on blood safety, universal precautions in clinical settings, the provision of condoms, and the dissemination of relevant information on prevention.

Other communicable diseases that have occurred in emergency or post-emergency settings have had a relatively minor impact. In the individual

setting in which they occur, however, they command an important allocation of resources and may be important contributors to morbidity and
mortality. Yellow fever, typhoid fever, relapsing fever, Japanese B encephali-
tis, dengue haemorrhagic fever, typhus, and leptospirosis are all real threats.
Nevertheless, morbidity and mortality has been shown time and again to be
due to the same conditions that are responsible for the bulk of the disease
burden in low-income countries in non-emergency settings.

Injuries

Injuries are widespread in all populations and are responsible for significant mortality, morbidity, and disability. Conflicts typically lead to substantial morbidity and mortality among civilians caused by a wide range
of weapons. Injuries, aside from those that are directly conflict-related, are
typically neglected in preference for an emphasis on communicable diseases. This is unfortunate given the widespread occurrence of intentional
(homicide, war, suicide) and unintentional (falls, traffic injuries, drowning,
poisoning) injuries in many populations affected by conflict. In situations
where injuries are shown to be major causes of morbidity and mortality,
they should be addressed as vigorously as communicable diseases and malnutrition.

Most attention has been focused on landmine injuries, an area in
which notable international successes have been achieved. Evidence of
the harmful effects of anti-personnel landmines and their concentration
in the world's poorest countries such as Angola, Ethiopia, Cambodia, and
Afghanistan, resulted in the Ottawa process that led to a ban on the production and distribution of anti-personnel mines. Aside from the direct
health problems associated with anti-personnel landmines, they create a
wide range of other problems—fear and insecurity—as well as limited
access to areas affected by mines which, consequently, become unavailable
for agriculture and animal husbandry. The long-term effects of landmines
are serious: high levels of surgical skill and resources are required and
repeated refitting and modification of prostheses are necessary if disability
is to be minimised.

Reproductive health

Unfortunately, reproductive health services for refugees and displaced
persons have often been considered to be secondary priorities. While

there is no doubt that the provision of food, water, sanitation, and shelter is the highest priority during a humanitarian emergency, steps should be taken to ensure that other critical health needs of women, men, and adolescents are met as quickly as possible.

Women are a particularly vulnerable subset of the population because the gender-based discrimination that is all too common in stable societies is frequently exacerbated in times of societal stress and meagre resources. Sexual violence against women has been well documented in a number of conflict settings as well as in some refugee camps. Uncontrolled violence and its aftermath are characterised by a number of specific features that impact negatively on reproductive health. These include the breakdown of family networks and the consequent loss of protection and safety, as well as channels of information to adolescents and women of reproductive age.

Loss of revenue within the family can result in a restricted ability to make appropriate reproductive health choices, and may predispose women and adolescents to risk through, for example, engagement in commercial sex work. Increased sole responsibility, as manifested by an increase in the proportion of female-headed households, also changes the way women spend their time and money as they seek increased security and well-being for their families. Finally, as with all members of the affected population, women tend to pay more attention to securing health services for life-saving interventions than for non-emergency reproductive health services.

A minimum initial package of essential reproductive health services has been developed and is recommended by the major relevant international agencies. They are described later in this chapter. Interventions beyond this essential package require major investments of time and personnel that should not be diverted from the principal task of reducing excessive preventable mortality as rapidly as possible. In all cases, special care must be taken to ensure that women heads of household are being given equitable quantities of food and non-food commodities for themselves and their families.

Mental health

War and political violence have direct and indirect mental health consequences for victims, relatives, neighbours, and communities. Anxiety, uncertainty, and fear about the future, and about whether family members and homesteads remain alive and intact, are a substantial cause of distress for affected individuals and communities. Among those who are forced to flee either as refugees or as internally displaced people, the lack of knowledge about relatives and property left behind cause stress and distress.

Despite ongoing challenges of maintaining lives and livelihoods, life as a refugee, especially in a camp situation, may be monotonous and conducive to stress, anxiety, and depression.

The extent of mental health 'trauma' experienced during and in the aftermath of war and conflict is controversial with some analysts identifying significant proportions of affected populations suffering from posttraumatic stress disorder, while others argue that this term and the response to it is medicalising an essentially social phenomenon. The former school calls for large-scale counselling and mental health support structures, while the latter argue that reconstituting a sense of community and humanity, and re-establishing livelihoods and community structures, are far more important interventions than trauma centres and counselling.

Public health priorities

Primary prevention

Primary prevention is the basic strategy of public health. The provision of adequate food, shelter, potable water, sanitation, and immunisation has proved problematic in low-income countries disrupted by war or overwhelmed by the influx of large numbers of refugees. Primary prevention in such circumstances, therefore, means stopping the violence, which is the root cause of refugee flows. More effective diplomatic and political mechanisms need to be developed that might resolve conflicts early in their evolution prior to the stage when food shortages occur, health services collapse, populations migrate, and significant adverse public health outcomes emerge. Although these initiatives are beyond the direct control of health practitioners, every opportunity should be taken to advocate for political solutions to the problems that are the root cause of population migration.

Secondary prevention

Secondary prevention is the domain of relief workers and agencies. It involves prevention of excess mortality and morbidity once a population migration has taken place. Upon arrival at their destination, refugees—most of whom tend to be women and children—may suffer severe anxiety or depression, compounded by the loss of dignity associated with complete dependence on the generosity of others for their survival. If refugee camps are located near borders or close to areas of continuing armed conflict, the desire for security is an overriding concern. Therefore, the first priority of any relief operation is to ensure adequate protection and camps should be placed sufficiently distant from borders to reassure refugees that they are safe.

To diminish the sense of helplessness and dependency, refugees should be given an active role in the planning and implementation of relief programs. Nevertheless, giving total control of the distribution of relief items to so-called refugee 'leaders' may be dangerous. For example, leaders of the former, Hutu-controlled Rwandan government took control of the distribution system in Zairian refugee camps in July 1994, resulting in relief supplies being diverted to young male members of the former Rwandan Army.

Basic needs

In the absence of conflict resolution, those communities that are totally dependent on external aid for their survival must be provided the basic minimum resources necessary to maintain health and well-being. The provision of adequate food, clean water, shelter, sanitation, and warmth will prevent the most severe public health consequences of complex emergencies. Public health priorities include a rapid needs assessment, the establishment of a health information system, measles vaccination, the control of diarrhoeal and other communicable diseases, maternal and child health services, and nutritional rehabilitation. Critical to the success of the response is coordination of the many agencies involved in the relief effort.

Information for action

The purposes of early rapid assessments are multiple. They can provide important information regarding the evolution of the refugee emergency, identify groups and areas at greatest risk, evaluate the existing local response capacity, determine the magnitude of external resources required, and indicate which health programs will be required in the short- and medium-term (Médecins sans Frontières and Epicentre 1999). After the response to an initial rapid assessment has been instituted, the development and implementation of ongoing health information systems immediately becomes a high priority activity.

Food and nutrition

In general, the goal of a refugee feeding program is to provide adequate quantities of nutrients through the general household distribution of food rations. General food rations should contain at least 2100 kilocalories of energy per person per day as well as the other essential nutrients (World Health Organisation 2000). Rations should take into consideration the demographic composition of the population, the climate, the specific needs of vulnerable groups, and access by the population to alternative sources of food and/or income. These rations should be provided to households and the equity of distribution needs to be carefully monitored. Experience has shown that women are fairer than men in distributing each food item in the correct quantity.

There may be population subgroups who either are already acutely malnourished or at high risk of becoming malnourished. These groups may require targeted feeding, or what is termed 'selective feeding', including food supplements for vulnerable groups and therapeutic feeding for the severely malnourished (World Health Organisation 2000).

Health services

In camp settings, health services should be organised to ensure that the major causes of morbidity and mortality are addressed through fixed facilities and outreach programs. An essential drug list and standardised treatment protocols are necessary elements of a curative program. Camp medical services need to ensure that women and children have preferential access and specific programs need to provide an integrated package of growth monitoring, immunisation, antenatal and postnatal care, the treatment of common ailments, and health promotion.

Refugee community health workers (CHW) are likely to understand the cultural, behavioural, and environmental influences on health status; contribute to a growing potential for self-care within the community; share the health service provision workload; build capacity and skills that will potentially be available after repatriation; and enhance the dignity of both the community and the health care providers themselves. CHWs who are relatively unskilled and trained within the community may be the mainstay of service provision. However, it is important to recognise that the presence of trained health workers within the affected community, whether these be traditional birth attendants (TBA), nurses, doctors, or others, represents an extremely valuable resource whose role should be facilitated in whatever services are developed with expatriate agency support.

Communicable disease control

Concern for the potential impact of communicable diseases has dominated the public health response in many refugee settings and has been frequently warranted. Although many of the technical interventions and public health programs used in emergencies draw heavily from their counterparts in stable settings, a few important differences should be considered. Most important among them include addressing the needs of the local, non-displaced, population; maintaining respect for national health policies when dealing with refugees; and promoting substantial community involvement as early as is feasible.

Because of the devastating impact that measles has had in many refugee emergencies, it has become almost universally accepted that mass measles vaccination, regardless of vaccination history or place of provenance, should be instituted as early during an emergency as possible. Leading reference publications accord measles immunisation the highest priority of all interventions and recommend that it be undertaken immediately after an initial rapid assessment regardless of the circumstances (Centers for Disease Control and Prevention 1992; Médecins sans Frontières 1997; Sphere Project 2000).

All health personnel should be sensitised to the potential impact of diarrhoea and should be skilled in most aspects of prevention and of treatment. The key to prevention lies in providing adequate sanitation facilities and at least the minimum recommended quantity of water of acceptable quality (Sphere Project 2000). The mainstay of diarrhoea case management is oral rehydration therapy. Rehydration facilities should be available in all health facilities, including health posts and outreach sites within the community. A key component of the program is preparedness planning for the control of cholera and dysentery outbreaks.

Given the high prevalence of HIV infection in many countries with large refugee populations, early attention should be given to HIV prevention (see the section below on reproductive health care).

Women's and children's health (WCH)

Health services oriented to the specific needs of children and women are essential in reducing morbidity and mortality within a population to a minimum level. WCH care should begin within the community, at the household level, and not depend entirely on established health facilities. For children, routine growth monitoring is an essential function of WCH services. A WCH program will also ensure that all children are vaccinated on schedule and are receiving regular supplements of vitamin A. Curative care, when required, can be offered at the household by trained CHWs or the child can be referred to health facilities.

All women should be vaccinated with tetanus toxoid to prevent neonatal tetanus in their newborn. Iron and folic acid should be distributed (and their ingestion monitored, if possible). Malaria chemoprophylaxis, if appropriate, should also be undertaken. In the post-natal period, counselling services should be offered addressing a variety of issues, from family planning to childcare, especially about breastfeeding.

Reproductive health care

Reproductive health care is among the crucial elements that give refugees the basic human welfare and dignity that is their right (UNHCR 1995). The response to reproductive health problems during emergencies consists of a constellation of assessment, services, and regular monitoring that addresses the implementation of the following programs:

- a minimum initial service package (MISP)
- safe motherhood
- prevention and treatment of sexual and gender-based violence
- prevention and care for sexually transmitted diseases
- family planning
- reproductive health needs of adolescents

The components of MISP have been described as follows:

Forced migration is frequently accompanied by sexual violence. To prevent unwanted pregnancies resulting from rape, emergency postcoital contraception supplies should be available to women who request them. Universal precautions to prevent the transmission of human immunodeficiency virus (HIV) must be respected from the very outset of an emergency. Although chaotic conditions are frequently prevalent and although health services are implemented under very stressful conditions, the threat of HIV infection can and must be minimised. To prevent unwanted pregnancies and to minimise the transmission of sexually transmitted infections, including AIDS, an adequate supply of condoms should be available on request to all members of the target population. In a population of 2500 with a crude birth rate of about 3 per cent, there will be five to eight births per month. In order to deal with these deliveries, simple supplies must be made available. Simple delivery kits and midwife kits are both readily available from UNICEF and other providers of health supplies.

The last element of the MISP is planning for the provision of comprehensive reproductive health services as rapidly as is feasible. To do this, reproductive health indicators should be included in health information systems to allow for the collection of baseline data on maternal, infant, and child mortality, prevalence of sexually transmitted diseases, and population contraceptive prevalence rates.

Conclusions

There are many non-governmental organisations (NGOs) engaged in providing humanitarian assistance to refugees and displaced persons; they include national Red Cross and Red Crescent societies, international secular and religious agencies, and local churches and community-based organisations in the affected country. The level of technical skills, experience, management, and logistics capacity of NGOs varies enormously. In an effort to promote coordination and best practice among NGOs, a number of initiatives have been taken. These include the Code of Conduct for the International Red Cross and Red Crescent Movement and NGOs in Disaster Response and the Humanitarian Charter and Minimum Standards in Disaster Response (Sphere Project 2000).

Significant progress has been made during the past two decades towards the provision of effective, focused, needs-based humanitarian assistance to conflict-affected populations. Greater emphasis is now placed on the impact, including health outcomes, of international aid. The quantity of aid delivered is no longer considered a valid indicator of effectiveness; its relevance, quality, coverage, and its equitable distribution are now accepted as more pertinent. As public health in refugee settings has developed as a specialised technical field, a number of relief agencies, especially NGOs, have developed technical manuals, field guidelines, and targeted training courses. Nevertheless, these initiatives will not be effective unless the international community adopts a more consistent approach to the early prevention and mitigation of conflict-related emergencies.

Recommended readings

Centers for Disease Control and Prevention (1992) Famine affected, refugee, and displaced populations: Recommendations for Public Health Issues, *MMWR Recommendations & Reports*, 41(RR–13): 1–76.

Médecins sans Frontières (1997) *Refugee Health: an approach to emergency situations,* Macmillan, London.

Sphere Project, The (2000) *Humanitarian Charter and Minimum Standards in Disaster Response*, The Sphere Project, Geneva.

Toole, M.J., Waldman, R.J. & Zwi, A. (2001) Complex Humanitarian Emergencies, In Merson, M., Black, R. & Mills, A. (eds), *Textbook of International Public Health. Diseases Programs, Systems and Policies*, Aspen Publications, Gaithersburg, Maryland, pp. 439–513.

References

Australian Department of Immigration and Multicultural and Indigenous Affairs (2001), available at: http://www.immi.gov.au.

Centers for Disease Control and Prevention (1991) Outbreak of pellagra among Mozambican refugees—Malawi, 1990, *MMWR*, 40: 209–13.

Centers for Disease Control and Prevention (1992) Famine affected, refugee, and displaced populations: Recommendations for Public Health Issues, *MMWR Recommendations & Reports,* 41(RR–13): 1–76.

Centers for Disease Control and Prevention (1993) Status of public health—Bosnia and Herzegovina, August–September 1993, *MMWR*, 42: 973, 979–82.

Desenclos, J.C., Berry, A.M., Padt, R., Farah, B., Segala, C. & Nabil, A.M. (1989) Epidemiologic patterns of scurvy among Ethiopian refugees, *Bulletin of the World Health Organization*, 67: 309–16.

Goma Epidemiology Group (1995) Public health impact of Rwandan refugee crisis. What happened in Goma, Zaïre, in July 1994, *Lancet*, 345: 339–44.

Médecins sans Frontières (1997) *Refugee Health: an approach to emergency situations,* Macmillan, London.

Médecins sans Frontières and Epicentre (1999) *Rapid health assessment of refugee or displaced populations*, MSF, Paris.

Sphere Project, The (2000) *Humanitarian Charter and Minimum Standards in Disaster Response*, Sphere Project, Geneva.

Toole, M. & Waldman, R. (1990) Prevention of excess mortality in refugee and displaced populations in developing countries, *Journal of the American Medical Association*, 263: 3296–3302.

Toole, M.J. & Bhatia, R. (1992) A case study of Somali refugees in Hartisheik A camp, eastern Ethiopia: health and nutrition profile, July 1988–June 1989, *Journal of Refugee Studies*, 5: 313–26.

Toole, M.J., Galson, S. & Brady, W. (1993) Are war and public health compatible? Report from Bosnia-Herzegovina, *Lancet*, 341: 1193–6.

Toole, M.J., Waldman, R.J. & Zwi, A. (2001) Complex Humanitarian Emergencies, In eds, Merson, M., Black, R. & Mills, A. (eds), *Textbook of International Public Health. Diseases Programs, Systems and Policies,* Aspen Publications, Gaithersburg, Maryland, pp. 439–513.

UNHCR (1995) *Reproductive health in refugee situations. An inter-agency field manual*, UNHCR, Geneva.

United States Committee for Refugees (1998) *World Refugee Survey 1998*, United States Committee for Refugees, Washington DC.

United States Committee for Refugees (2001) *World Refugee Survey 2001*, United States Committee for Refugees, Washington DC.

World Health Organisation (1999), Health Situation Report-East Timor, In Health Information Network for Advanced Planning (HINAP).

World Health Organisation (2000) *The management of nutrition in major emergencies*, World Health Organisation, Geneva.

Yip, R. & Sharp, T.W. (1993) Acute malnutrition and high childhood mortality related to diarrhea, *Journal of the American Medical Association*, 270: 587–90.

4

Refugee Health: Clinical Issues

Beverley-Ann Biggs and Susan A. Skull

Introduction

Many refugees have reached Australia after a long and arduous journey, often involving months or years in refugee camps and exposure to traumatic events including physical hardship and illness. Refugees and immigrants often come from parts of the world where endemic diseases differ to those in Australia and access to health care is poor. In particular, parasitic and tropical diseases may be inadequately treated, chronic diseases may have been poorly managed, and immunisation may be incomplete. On arrival in Australia, settlers face the challenges of difficult economic circumstances, cultural and language barriers, and separation from family and friends.

Recent figures show that nearly one in four of Australia's current population of 18.7 million is overseas born. Studies suggest that people with refugee-like experiences have a higher rate of long-term medical and psychological conditions, have a poorer state of well-being and visit health care providers more frequently (Lehn 1997). There is therefore an urgent need to examine and strengthen health services to ensure optimal health in settlers and to monitor the prevalence of communicable and non-communicable diseases. This chapter will focus on some of the clinical issues that are of special concern to immigrants and refugees. The information presented should be utilised in the context of a holistic approach to health that recognises the wide variation within and between immigrant groups from different countries and regions.

Refugee trends in Australia

In Australia a marked increase occurred in the number of refugees and migrant arrivals from Vietnam, Cambodia, and Laos in the late 1970s and 1980s, due to conflict in Indo-China and changes in Australian immigration policy (Goldstein et al. 1987). During the period 1974 to 1991 approximately 150,000 South-East Asian refugees and migrants resettled in Australia, predominantly in the states of New South Wales and Victoria.

Since 1991 Australia's Humanitarian Program has focused largely on people from the former Yugoslavia, the Middle East, and the Horn of Africa. This is illustrated in figure 4.1. Ninety-two per cent of Humanitarian Program entrants from Africa come from Somalia, Sudan, Ethiopia, Eritrea, and Kenya. These people are likely to have suffered extreme hardship due to conflict and war in their country of origin and have often spent extended periods in prisons and camps with poor sanitation, little access to safe drinking water and food, psychological and physical abuse, overcrowding and intermittent or incomplete health services (Victorian Foundation for the Survivors of Torture 2002). Similarly, people arriving from Bosnia-Herzegovina, Iran, and Iraq may have experienced harsh conditions and poor access to health care.

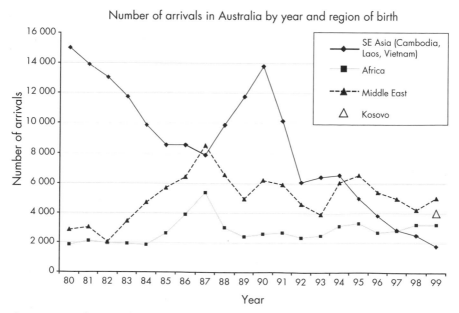

Figure 4.1 Refugee and immigrant intake in Australia since 1982
Source: Department of Immigration and Multicultural and Indigenous Affairs

Australia provided a temporary safe haven for nearly 4000 Kosovar refugees in 1999 in the largest single humanitarian evacuation ever undertaken in Australia. Difficulties in establishing and maintaining health surveillance and monitoring systems, and the further intake of refugees from East Timor in that year, highlight the need for preparedness in dealing with refugee health crises (Bennett et al. 2000), see also (Smith & Harvey p. 139).

Most people with 'refugee-like' experiences enter Australia through the Refugee and Special Humanitarian Program. This program includes refugees as well as those who have close family or community links in Australia and who are in vulnerable situations in their country of origin. People from similar backgrounds may also enter through other Australian migration programs, and immigrants and refugees are collectively known as settlers. Settlers from developing countries may experience the same health problems whatever their category of entry and these relate to poverty and inadequate health care.

Screening and health assessments

Refugee and migrant screening clinics were established in the 1970s to assess and manage the health of refugees and immigrants from South-East Asia, including immunisation, chronic disease and infectious diseases such as intestinal parasite infections, tuberculosis, hepatitis B and sexually transmitted diseases. In Victoria alone, approximately 50,000 South-East Asian refugees and migrants were screened between 1974 and 1991 (McKay 1991). In retrospect, screening was considered to be neither universal nor particularly effective as many individuals had no pathology or only visited a clinic once and had inadequate or no follow-up (McKay 1991). There was also the perception that the cost of screening outweighed the public health benefits, as there was no demonstrated risk of spread of communicable diseases to the broader Australian community (Goldstein et al. 1987).

Currently, doctors nominated by the Australian Government undertake limited pre-arrival screening for all entrants before departure from the country of origin. A medical examination is performed and tests undertaken as shown in table 4.1. Serious infectious diseases such as tuberculosis (TB) are treated prior to arrival.

Emergency refugees who are evacuated at short notice (such as the Kosovars and East Timorese in recent times, see chapter nine) do not necessarily undergo orderly pre-arrival screening. Following pre-arrival health screening, some entrants will be asked to sign a health undertaking that they will contact the Commonwealth Health Undertaking Service for follow-up monitoring. The majority of people on a health undertaking are

Table 4.1 Health checks for people wanting to migrate to Australia

Pre-arrival Screening Test	Recipient
Chest X-ray (TB)	All applicants > 16 years, or younger if there are indications they have TB or have a history of contact with a person with TB
HIV serology	All applicants >15 years International adoptees History of blood transfusions or other clinical indications
HBV serology	Pregnant women International adoptees Unaccompanied refugee minors
Syphilis serology (VDRL)	Applicants at risk of STDs Applicants > 16 years who have lived in refugee-camp-like conditions
Urinalysis	All applicants > 5 years
Height and Weight	All applicants

Source. Department of Immigration and Multicultural and Indigenous Affairs, notes for Guidance of Overseas Panel Doctors, Radiologists, Commonwealth Medical Officers, Approved Medical Practitioners, and Migration Officers on the Health Assessment of Visa Applicants, Canberra, 1999.

those who are pre-identified as having or possibly having TB. Individual states and territories are responsible for all other post-arrival health care of settlers. While the extent of formal post-arrival health screening or assessment varies between states and serritories, in many areas immigrant and refugee health has become the responsibility of medical practitioners at the primary health care level. At present, some states such as Victoria have no formal post-arrival health care process that links primary health providers with new immigrants, but emphasis is being placed on strengthening existing immigrant health resources and networks (Billi 1999).

Specific medical conditions

The utilisation of health care services by settlers may not be optimal especially within the first few months of arrival. Literacy problems and cultural differences in health-seeking behaviour may be important barriers to the use of health services, as well as limited services linking new arrivals into the Australian health care system. In addition, health services may be ill prepared to deal with cultural and language differences and unusual disease patterns. Infectious diseases are of particular importance as they are endemic in many developing countries and may cause illness in immigrants and refugees after resettlement. Mental health, dental health, and chronic illness also impart a high burden of often-unrecognised disease.

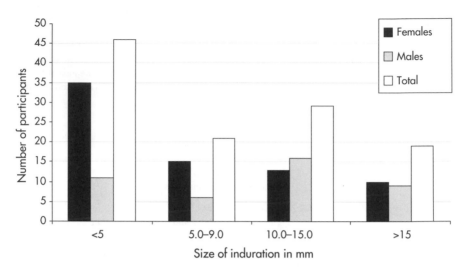

Figure 4.2 Distribution of Mantoux test results in recently arrived adult settlers from East Africa

Some important examples of communicable and non-communicable diseases for consideration in this group are highlighted below.

Communicable diseases

Tuberculosis

TB is a potentially life-threatening infection that is endemic in many developing countries. Initial infection is often asymptomatic, with the risk of progression to symptomatic disease increasing with age. Inactive (latent) infection may be detected with a Mantoux test and, in those aged 35 years or less, preventative treatment is usually recommended. One of the periods of greatest risk for developing symptomatic disease is in the first few years after immigration to a new country (MacIntyre & Plant 1998). Currently, persons with a normal chest X-ray prior to departure for Australia are not followed for the development of TB after arrival, and it is not known what proportion of immigrants have latent TB infection. However, recently arrived immigrants diagnosed with TB constitute a considerable number of those currently being treated for TB in tertiary hospitals (see figure 4.2) and it has been suggested that many cases may be prevented with updated guidelines and better implementation of early detection and treatment policy (MacIntyre & Plant 1998).

HIV diagnoses, 1994–2000, by exposure category

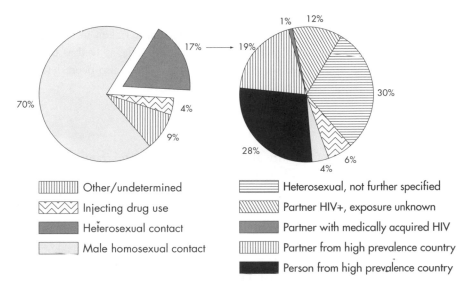

▨ Other/undetermined		▦ Heterosexual, not further specified	
▧ Injecting drug use		▨ Partner HIV+, exposure unknown	
▨ Heterosexual contact		▨ Partner with medically acquired HIV	
▨ Male homosexual contact		▦ Partner from high prevalence country	
		■ Person from high prevalence country	

Figure 4.3 HIV diagnosis in settlers who have migrated from countries with high transmission rates
Source: National Centre in HIV Epidemiology and Clinical Research, http://www.med.unsw.edu.au/nchecr/default.htm

HIV/AIDS

Some refugees originate from countries in which HIV infection is highly endemic. Pre-arrival HIV testing is a prerequisite for all adult immigrants but individuals may test negative in the early stages of infection and may be exposed later during home visits. In the period 1994–99 exposure to HIV was attributed to heterosexual contact in 17 per cent of new diagnoses in Australia. Close to half of these cases were in people from countries with high HIV prevalence (figure 4.3). Early diagnosis of HIV infection is paramount, as intervention with antiretroviral drugs will significantly delay the onset of ill health and AIDS and reduce HIV transmission. This is particularly important for infected women of childbearing age prior to conception.

Other sexually transmitted infections

The prevalence of sexually transmitted infections (STIs) is higher in developing countries. In addition, refugees and immigrants may have suffered sexual violence and exploitation in their own country or in refugee camps en route to Australia. The prevalence of syphilis in settlers who entered Australia from Asia, Africa, and Central and South America varied from 4 per cent to 10 per cent in a screening program undertaken in Victoria in the 1980s (McKay 1991). Gonorrhoea and chlamydia, as well as tropical STDs such as granuloma inguinale (donovanosis) have also been detected in recent arrivals.

Hepatitis B

The prevalence of hepatitis B (HB) infection in immigrants from Asia, Africa, and Oceania is between 12 per cent and 22 per cent. HB also has significant health implications for the individual, as chronic infection results in chronic hepatitis, cirrhosis, and/or hepatocellular carcinoma in up to one third of affected individuals. Chronic infection is most likely to result after exposure at birth or in the first five years of life. Therefore, universal immunisation of all infants against HB is recommended (National Health and Medical Research Council (Australia) 2000).

In a recent study of Laotian refugees who had been settled in Victoria for an average of 12 years, 9/95 (9 per cent) of adults had chronic HB infection. Seven of these were previously undiagnosed (S. DeSilva, personal communication). Similarly, surveys of adult East African immigrants to Victoria in 2000–01 found that 7/123 (6 per cent) adults and 2/108 (2 per cent) children had chronic HB infection, of whom only one was previously aware of their diagnosis (Ngeow 2000).

It is important that individuals with chronic HB infection are identified in order to provide information about transmissibility, immunisation of family members and partners, as well as to ensure appropriate management of the complications of chronic HB infection if and when they arise.

Hepatitis C

The number of reported cases of hepatitis C (HC) continues to rise globally. High risk groups include injecting drug users and some groups in developing countries have a higher background prevalence of HC, possibly because of the past use of improperly sterilised medical equipment. HC poses similar risks to HB with up to 80 per cent of infected persons becoming chronic carriers. A significant proportion will progress to chronic hepatitis, cirrhosis, and/or hepatocellular carcinoma.

Parasitic diseases

Intestinal parasite infections cause a major disease burden in most developing countries. It is therefore not surprising that they are the most prevalent communicable diseases occurring in immigrants and refugees (Cantanzaro & Moser 1982; Gyorkos et al. 1989; Molina et al. 1998; Nutman et al. 1987). The prevalence of parasitic infections has been found to be as high as 30 per cent to 50 per cent in newly arrived adult settlers from Indo-China (Gyorkos et al. 1992; Hoffman et al. 1981; Lindes 1979; Ryan et al. 1988). Recent Victorian surveys have found significant evidence of that pathogenic parasitic infection on faecal microscopy in migrants from Laos and children and adults from East Africa (De Silva et al. 2002; Ngeow 2000). Although easily treated with short course oral medication, infections are often undetected because symptoms can be low grade and chronic.

Strongyloides stercoralis infection may persist for decades, causing recurrent skin rash and abdominal pain, and occasionally life-threatening disseminated infection in those who become immuno-compromised (Genta 1989; Grove 1996; Lim & Biggs 2001; Sampson & Grove 1987). Strongyloidiasis has been confirmed as a particular problem in some groups of South-East Asian immigrants (Gyorkos et al. 1990) and a 23 per cent point prevalence of chronic *S. stercoralis* infection was found in adult Laotian immigrants in Victoria (De Silva et al. 2002). See table 4.2.

Similarly, schistosomiasis may appear years after resettlement and result in serious complications. The East African surveys found rates of positive or equivocal serology in 12 per cent of adults and 2 per cent of children (Ngeow 2000). Malaria may occur in settlers from endemic areas especially Africa (Robinson et al. 2001) and should be excluded in presentations of fever as *Plasmodium falciparum* malaria may be fatal.

Incomplete immunisation

While many countries have vaccination programs in place, geographic isolation or disruption of health services due to political and social instability may result in an incomplete vaccination status. Furthermore, new immigrants may arrive without any documentation of previous vaccinations. Two surveys conducted among East African adult and paediatric settlers in Victoria in 2001–02 found that documentation of vaccination status was absent for most and the majority were unable to recall which vaccinations they had previously received. Furthermore, based on serological evidence, recall was often found to be unreliable (Ngeow 2000).

Table 4.2 Frequency of organisms detected in recent and long-term adult and paediatric settlers by stool microscopy (wet preparation and/or faecal concentration of a single specimen) or serology

Organisms[a]	South-East Asian Adults[b] (n = 87) (%)	East African Adults (n = 117) (%)	East African Children (n = 133) (%)
Pathogens			
Giardia lamblia	1 (1)	6 (5)	7(5)
Entamoeba histolytica/dispar		4 (3)	5 (4)
Ankylostoma spp.	2 (2)		5 (4)
Trichuris trichiura		5 (4)	3 (2)
Strongyloides stercoralis	2 (2)		
S. stercoralis (serology positive)	22 (23)[c]		1
Opisthorcis spp.	3 (3)		
Hymenolepis nana		1 (1)	5 (4)
Schistosoma mansoni	ND		1 (1)
Schistosoma spp. (serology positive)	ND	14 (12)	3 (2)
Non-pathogens		104	96
Blastocystis homini[d]	3 (3)	51 (44)	39 (29)
Iodamoeba butschlii		3 (3)	5 (4)
Entamoeba coli		22 (19)	25 (19)
Endolimax nana		26 (22)	19 (14)
Entamoeba hartmanni		1 (1)	5 (4)
Chilomastix mesnili		0 (0)	3 (2)
Dientamoeba fragilis[d]		1 (1)	3 (2)

a.   More than one organism detected per participant in some cases.
b.   A wet preparation was not examined in the Laotian group.
c.   N = 95.
d.   Occasionally pathogenic and symptomatic patients should be treated.

Serology results indicated that inadequate immunity was present in 80 per cent of children for at least one of tetanus, diphtheria, measles, hepatitis B (no HbsAb or HbcAb detected), or rubella. While most adults had immunity to measles, overall, 100 (81 per cent) had inadequate immunity to at least one of measles, tetanus, hepatitis B, and diphtheria (see table 4.3).

It is also important to note many vaccines on the Australian Standard Vaccination Schedule are not universally available (for example *Haemo-*

Table 4.3 Levels of inadequate immunity to vaccine-preventable diseases among East African adults and children in Victoria as proven by serological survey

Inadequate Immunity	Children (%)	Adults (%)
Tetanus	42/98 (43)	82/123 (67)
Diphtheria	57/100 (57)	42/123 (34)
Measles	13/90 (14)	4/123 (3)
Hepatitis B	64/100 (64)	50/123 (41)
Rubella	23/98 (23)	—
For at least one of the above	78/98 (80)	100/123 (81)

philus influenzae B and hepatitis B vaccines) and additional vaccinations may be required.

Non-communicable diseases

Vitamin D and other nutritional deficiencies

Vitamin D is essential for skeletal health, and severe deficiency is associated with defective mineralisation resulting in rickets in children and osteomalacia in adults. These conditions can result in growth abnormalities and fractures due to brittle bones. Dark pigmentation and reduced sunlight exposure present risk factors of vitamin D deficiency and disease may be asymptomatic until an advanced stage. A recent Australian study showed that Caucasian women are at risk of vitamin D deficiency in Victoria (latitude 38 degrees south), with rates of over 10 per cent recorded in Geelong in winter (Pasco et al. 2001). For dark skinned immigrant groups, women who remain largely covered for religious reasons and those who may have had restricted sun exposure due to conflict and other refugee experiences, the effects of low sun exposure can be particularly dramatic. In 2001 Nozza and Rodda reported that 54/55 children with vitamin D deficiency were born to mothers with ethno-cultural risk factors for vitamin D deficiency. The majority (81 per cent) of these mothers who were tested were also vitamin D deficient (Nozza & Rodda 2001). In addition, Grover and Morley (2001) reported that 80 per cent of dark skinned or veiled women attending a Melbourne antenatal clinic had vitamin D deficiency (Grover & Morley 2001).

Other nutritional deficiencies, including iron, thiamine, iodine, and vitamin C, may occur in refugees, especially those spending long periods in camps (Mason 2002). Patients with anaemia in whom micronutrient deficiency has been excluded should also be assessed for a red blood cell disorder, such as thalassaemia and sickle cell anaemia.

Mental health

Refugees entering under the Humanitarian Program are likely to have had traumatic experiences in, or during their flight from their countries of origin, and may be experiencing associated physical and psychological sequelae (Victorian Foundation for the Survivors of Torture 2002). These include post-traumatic stress disorder, depression, anxiety, psychosis, dissociation and somatic disorders (Keyes 2000). Traumatic effects on children also have been described, including withdrawal, fear, aggression and somatic complaints (Gavagan & Brodyaga 1998). Many children have witnessed violence to family members or have themselves been victims of violence. Health professionals seeing refugees need to orient their consultation and management to accommodate the negative effects of reaction to past trauma, prior experience of health care, cultural differences, and the stresses of resettlement. Referral to appropriate mental health services or community support groups may be necessary.

Other conditions

Insulin dependent diabetes mellitus (IDDM) is a chronic disorder with high morbidity. Early recognition, treatment, and education are necessary to minimise complications. There is evidence that some immigrant populations have high rates of IDDM, for example Asian immigrants to the United Kingdom (Kibirige 1999), perhaps related to changes in diet or lifestyle. In addition, diabetes may be unrecognised in the early phases and there may be difficulties in accessing health care.

Assessment of dental health is particularly important in refugee patients as there may have been limited access to dental care services, poor diet, or injuries sustained.

Cancer screening may be required according to age-appropriate guidelines, and clinicians should be particularly alert for cancer types that occur with increased frequency in other parts of the world. These cancer types include gastric, lung (as cigarette smoking expands globally) and hepatocellular carcinoma (resulting from hepatitis B infection). Cervical cancer is more frequent in some countries because of infrequent or absent pap screening programs (Gavagan & Brodyaga 1998). The timing of screening will depend on whether or not the patient is symptomatic and should take into account that invasive screening procedures may be distressing. In many cases it may be appropriate to delay screening until a relationship of trust is established between patient and doctor (Victorian Foundation for the Survivors of Torture 2002).

Summary

In the last two decades Australia has experienced several waves of migration and accepted thousands of refugees. Refugees and immigrants from developing countries have special health needs as they are at increased risk from infectious diseases such as TB, HIV, viral hepatitis, parasitic diseases, as well as incomplete immunisations, psychological and other physical health problems such as dental disease, vitamin D and other nutritional deficiencies, and chronic diseases. Language and cultural barriers often prevent these settlers accessing or even being aware of available health care services in Australia. In some states, the establishment of local refugee health services to replace the mass refugee health screening programs of the 1970s and 1980s has tried to address this. However, the challenge now is to establish a consistent nationwide network of health services to cater for the special needs of refugees and immigrants, regardless of entry category. This will require close consultation with settlers, health providers, and public health stakeholders as well as a program of ongoing education to raise awareness of health needs among community members.

Acknowledgments

We thank Sabine De Silva, Dr Joanne Ngeow, Dr Pao Saykao, Dr Jonathan Carapetis, Dr James Rice, Dr George McGillivray, Western Region Health Centre, Banyule Community Health Service, the South-East Asian and East African communities and others involved in the studies conducted by the authors and referred to in this chapter. We also thank Graham Brown, Alan Street, Daniel O'Brien, Kim Webster, Sonia Caruana and John Carnie for helpful suggestions and Virginia de Crespigny for assistance with the manuscript. Our work has been supported by the University of Melbourne, the Victorian Infectious Diseases Service at the Royal Melbourne Hospital, the Department of Paediatrics at the Royal Children's Hospital, the Victorian Infectious Diseases Reference Laboratory, the Victorian Foundation for the Survivors of Torture, and the Department of Human Services.

Recommended reading

Billi, R. (1999) *Refugee health-screening and assessment. Protocols and Practices—an Australian Perspective 1999*, Victorian Public Health Training Scheme, Department of Human Services Victoria, Melbourne.

Victorian Foundation for the Survivors of Torture (2002) *Promoting refugee health—a handbook for doctors and other health care providers caring for people from refugee backgrounds*, VFST Inc., Melbourne.

References

Bennett, C., Mein, J., Beers, M., Harvey, B., Vemeulpad, S., Chant, K. & Dalton, C. (2000) Operation Safe Haven: an evaluation of health surveillance and monitoring in an acute setting, *Communicable Diseases Intelligence*, 24: 1–7.

Billi, R. (1999) *Refugee health-screening and assessment. Protocols and Practices—an Australian Perspective 1999*, Victorian Public Health Training Scheme, Department of Human Services Victoria, Melbourne.

Cantanzaro, A. & Moser, R.J. (1982) Health status of refugees from Vietnam, Laos, and Cambodia, *Journal of the American Medical Association*, 242: 1303–8.

De Silva, S., Saykao, P., Kelly, H., MacIntyre, C.R., Ryan, N., Leydon, J. & Biggs, B.A. (2002) Chronic *Strongyloides stercoralis* infection in the Laotian refugee population seven to twenty years after resettlement in Australia, *Epidemiology and infection*, 128(3): 439–44.

Gavagan, T. & Brodyaga, L. (1998) Medical care for immigrants and refugees, *American Family Physician*, 57(5): 1061–8.

Genta, R.M. (1989) Global prevalence of strongyloidiasis: critical review with epidemiologic insights into the prevention of disseminated disease, *Review of Infectious Diseases*, 11: 755–67.

Goldstein, G.B., Reid, J.C. & Keo, L. (1987) A review of refugee medical screening in New South Wales, *Medical Journal of Australia*, 146: 9–12.

Grove, D.I. (1996) Human strongyloidiasis, *Advances in Parasitology*, 38: 251–309.

Grover, S.R. & Morley, R. (2001) Vitamin D deficiency in veiled or dark-skinned pregnant women, *Medical Journal of Australia*, 175: 251–52.

Gyorkos, T.W., Frappier-Davignon, L., MacLean, J.D. & Viens, P. (1989) Effect of screening and treatment on imported intestinal parasite infections: results from a randomized, controlled trial, *American Journal of Epidemiology*, 129: 753–61.

Gyorkos, T.W., Genta, R.M., Viens, P. & MacLean, J.D. (1990) Seroepidemiology of Strongyloides infection in the Southeast Asian refugee population in Canada, *American Journal of Epidemiology*, 132: 257–64.

Gyorkos, T.W., MacLean, J.D., Viens, P., Cheang, C. & Kokoskin-Nelson, E. (1992) Intestinal parasite infection in the Kampuchean refugee population 6 years after resettlement in Canada, *Journal of Infectious Diseases*, 166: 413–17.

Hoffman, S.L., Barrett-Connor, E., Norcross, W. & Nguyen, D. (1981) Intestinal parasites in Indochinese immigrants, *The American Journal of Tropical Medicine & Hygiene*, 30: 340–3.

Keyes, E.F. (2000) Mental health status in refugees: an integrative review of current research, *Issues in Mental Health Nursing*, 21(4): 397–410.

Kibirige, M.S. (1999) Diabetes in immigrant Asian children, *Indian Pediatrics*, 36(5): 445–8.

Lehn, A. (1997) Recent immigrants' health and their utilisation of medical services. Results from the longitudinal survey of immigrants to Australia, *Department of Immigration and Multicultural and Indigenous Affairs Immigration Update 1997*, March Quarter: 32–8.

Lim, L.L. & Biggs, B.A. (2001) Fatal disseminated strongyloidiasis in a previously screened and treated patient, *Medical Journal of Australia*, 174(7): 355–6.

Lindes, C. (1979) Intestinal Parasites in Laotian Refugees, *Journal of Family Practice*, 9: 819–22.

MacIntyre, C.R. & Plant, A.J. (1998) Tuberculosis in South-East Asian refugees after resettlement—can prevention be improved by better policy and practice, *Preventive Medicine*, 27: 815–20.

Mason, J. (2002) Lessons on nutrition of displaced people, *Journal of Nutrition*, 132(Supplement): 2096–2103.

McKay, S.R. (1991) *Refugee/Migrant Screening in Victoria*, Health Department Victoria, Melbourne.

Molina, C.D., Molina, M. & Molina, J.M. (1998) Intestinal parasites in Southeast Asian refugees two years after immigration, *Western Journal of Medicine*, 149: 422–5.

National Health and Medical Research Council (Australia) (2000) *The Australian immunisation handbook*, NHMRC, Canberra.

Ngeow, J.Y.Y. (2000) Assessment of the health and vaccination status of recently-arrived East African immigrants, BMedSci thesis, University of Melbourne, Melbourne.

Nozza, J.M. & Rodda, C.P. (2001) Vitamin D deficiency in mothers of infants with rickets, *Medical Journal of Australia*, 175: 253–5.

Nutman, T.B., Ottesen, E.A., Ieng, S., et al. (1987) Eosinophilia in Southeast Asian refugees: evaluation at a referral center, *Journal of Infectious Diseases*, 155: 309–13.

Pasco, J.A., Henry, M.J., Nicholson, G.C., Sanders, K.M. & Kotowicz, M.A. (2001) Vitamin D status of women in the Geelong Osteoporosis Study: association with diet and casual exposure to sunlight, *Medical Journal of Australia*, 175(8): 401–5.

Robinson, P., Jenney, A.W., Tachado, M., Yung, A., Manitta, J., Taylor, K. & Biggs, B.A. (2001) Imported malaria treated in Melbourne, Australia: epidemiology and clinical features in 246 patients, *Journal of Travel Medicine*, 8(2): 76–81.

Ryan, N.M., Plackett, M. & Dwyer, B. (1988) Parasitic infections of refugees, *Medical Journal of Australia*, 148: 491–4.

Sampson, I.A. & Grove, D.I. (1987) Strongyloidiasis is endemic in another Australian population group: Indochinese immigrants, *Medical Journal of Australia*, 146: 580–2.

Victorian Foundation for the Survivors of Torture (2002) *Promoting refugee health—a handbook for doctors and other health care providers caring for people from refugee backgrounds*, VFST Melbourne.

5

Mental Health of Asylum Seekers: Australia in a Global Context

Derrick Silove

In the last decade there has been a progressive deterioration in the way asylum seekers have been treated when seeking refuge in developed countries of the West. In countries such as Australia that have a quota for refugee intake, an increasingly sharp distinction has been made between 'offshore' refugees who successfully lodge applications outside the country, and asylum seekers who arrive without valid resettlement documents. The asylum seeker group live under increasingly stringent restrictions and deprivations while awaiting the outcomes of their refugee claims, with special concerns being focused on those held in immigration detention centres (Steel & Silove 2001; Sultan & O'Sullivan 2001).

Although detention is used on a discretionary basis in other Western countries, Australia stands alone in mandating the automatic detention of all persons arriving without valid entry documents, irrespective of the strength of their refugee claims. In 2001, the Australian Government also initiated an unprecedented strategy, the so-called 'Pacific Plan', in which naval intervention has been used to divert boatloads of asylum seekers to neighbouring island states in the Pacific region. Thus, Australia represents a special case in its management of asylum seekers, yet the impact of that country's policy on the psychosocial well-being of asylum issues is of global relevance since there is a risk that other Western countries may feel encouraged to pursue similarly restrictive approaches.

In this chapter, I outline briefly the historical background to the present asylum crisis in Australia, as a prelude to reviewing evidence relating to the mental health and psychosocial consequences of contemporary policies. In exploring these issues, I examine what might be referred to as the grand fallacies about asylum seekers: that most of them are not genuine refugees but unscrupulous intruders or hapless victims of people smugglers; that the way they are being treated in countries such as Australia is humane; that their administrative management is not injurious to their mental health; and that their protest actions, particularly when in detention, indicate a lack of integrity and/or a deliberate flouting of the laws and customs of the host country. I conclude by contrasting contemporary principles underlying the fields of human rights, mental health promotion and social development, with the actualities of the way asylum seekers are treated, in order to highlight the growing and unsustainable contradictions in the treatment of survivors of mass conflict and displacement seeking asylum in Western countries.

Historical background

The Refugee Convention, established in 1951 and extended by the Protocol of 1967, enshrined the right of persons fleeing from persecution to seek protection in signatory countries. Implicit in the spirit of the convention was an international undertaking to treat persons escaping oppressive regimes in a dignified and respectful manner, and to take reasonable steps to provide for their human needs. The tragic consequences of the Nazi Holocaust undoubtedly were a major driving force behind the formulation and adoption of the convention. The genocide provided a stark lesson to Western countries about the potential for disaster when early signs of mass persecution are ignored. Thus, underpinning the convention was a fundamental commitment to ensure that the world community would never again fail to offer humane and dignified protection to those who are unjustly victimised for political, ideological, religious, and other beliefs, and who are faced with no other choice but to flee their homelands to evade persecution.

The Cold War strengthened the spirit of the convention since there was a broad-based consensus in Western countries that persons fleeing from totalitarian regimes were champions of democracy and freedom—heroes that neatly matched the public image of the genuine political refugee. Changes to this perception gained ground during the 1970s, particularly with the egress of hundreds of thousands of persons from South-East Asia at the conclusion of the war in Vietnam (Grant 1979), the accession of the Pol Pot regime in Cambodia (Mollica et al. 1993), and the communist takeover in Laos. The sheer volume of the populations crossing national borders over a short space of time had no precedence since World War II, the groups were of non-European origin, and the confusion surrounding the effective defeat of the US-led military intervention in Vietnam created ambivalence about the obligations of Western countries to provide further assistance to peoples from that region.

Although thousands of South-East Asians were accepted into Western countries during the early waves of flight, as the flow continued there was a greater resistance to accepting more refugees, and large numbers became sequestrated in neighbouring countries of first asylum, themselves developing countries with limited resources (Grant 1979). International agencies, such as the United Nations High Commissioner for Refugees (UNHCR) were ill-prepared to deal with such a large and complex flow of displaced persons. Conditions in refugee camps were often poor, administrative responsibility for displaced persons was ambiguous, and the ultimate fate of these populations remained uncertain for protracted periods of time (Mollica et al. 1993). The widespread use of the refugee camp and, in locations such as Hong Kong, of detention centres, signalled an important turning point in contemporary refugee policies; the introduction of a strategy in which confinement, restriction, separation from the host society, and extensive screening procedures were implemented in dealing with refugee flows.

Since then, refugee camps have proliferated in Africa, the Middle East, and various parts of Asia; most commonly in states bordering conflict-ridden countries in which solutions to inter-ethnic wars remain elusive. Some camps, such as Kakuma Camp in north-western Kenya (Silove & Ekblad 1998) have remained operational for decades, with many becoming a de facto home for long-term inhabitants. In some camps, children and adolescents have known no experience other than life in the camp.

In the last decade of the twentieth century, a further milestone in refugee policy occurred; the extension of the model of confinement to Western countries with the introduction of the asylum detention centre (Silove et al. 1993). Prior to this time, traditional refugee recipient countries such as Canada, the USA, and Australia accepted quotas of refugees, almost all of whom were screened and authorised 'offshore' by UN agencies or embassy staff in foreign countries. Even then, selection biases became increasingly evident with only a small minority of eligible applicants being resettled in Western countries. Over time, as numbers in refugee camps increased, the likelihood of being accepted for permanent resettlement in Western recipient countries progressively declined. In other instances, for example in Iraq, and in Afghanistan during the Taliban rule, the cessation of consular ties prevented vulnerable persons from applying for asylum 'offshore'. The consequence of all these pressures has been an overall increase in persons travelling by whatever means they are able to gain access to Western countries where they then seek asylum. Hence, persons under threat in countries such as Iraq, Afghanistan, Iran, and Sri Lanka often have no choice but to obtain falsified documents and to place their faith in underground networks of 'people smugglers' in order to reach a situation of safety.

Political representations of asylum seekers

Yet, the desperate measures asylum seekers use to achieve refuge have been increasingly utilised by governments and politicians in the West to cast doubt on their integrity and on the validity of their claims for protection. In Australia, asylum seekers are accused of being 'queue jumpers' who displace 'genuine' refugees from the intake quota; boat people have been publicly accused of setting boats alight and of throwing their children overboard; and the inference has been drawn that asylum groups may be harbouring terrorists within their midst. None of these assertions has been supported by evidence, and, in some instances, the opposite has been proven (for example, videotapes have shown asylum seekers holding infant children above the rails of boats to indicate that young persons were on board, rather than, as accused, that parents were trying to throw their children overboard). Nevertheless, there seems little doubt that the public in countries like Australia are now confused and polarised in their perceptions of asylum seekers.

Research into the plight of asylum seekers in Australia

Some light can be thrown on the true nature of the asylum population by examining salient characteristics that are relevant both to their mental health status and their refugee claims. Important indicators are the level of exposure to past abuses and the occurrence of particular patterns of psychological reactions that are known to be outcomes of such experiences. The base for comparison has been provided by a growing number of epidemiological studies undertaken among diverse populations of displaced persons worldwide (Mollica et al. 1993; Shrestha et al. 1998; Van Ommeren et al. 2001). Cross-cultural assessment tools have been developed and applied, allowing objective comparisons to be made across contexts in relation to the type and range of trauma suffered (Mollica et al. 1987), and the patterns of stress reactions that manifest among survivors. Although there is some variation in findings, depending on culture, ethnicity, and the nature of the conflict from which populations have fled (de Jong et al. 2001), the broad pattern of results remains consistent: displaced populations include substantial numbers of persons who have suffered torture, political harassment, and a wide range of related abuses and deprivations. Also, consistently, these populations include persons with trauma-related mental health sequelae including depression, post-traumatic stress disorder (PTSD) and anxiety (de Jong et al. 2001; Mollica et al. 1993). The more severe the trauma exposure, the greater the risk of adverse mental health outcomes (Mollica et al. 1993), and some forms of trauma, particularly torture, are demonstrably damaging to future psychosocial adaptation (Van Ommeren et al. 2001). Most importantly, the quality of the post-migration environment plays a significant role in determining the outcome of pre-existing traumatic stress reactions—the more insecure, threatening, and restrictive the conditions are, the more likely it is that symptoms will persist and become disabling (Silove & Kinzie 2001).

Do asylum seeker populations show similar trauma-related characteristics?

Research with asylum seekers to identify trauma related characteristics has been challenging: they are thinly dispersed in the population, there are no registers or other systematic methods for gathering epidemiological data on this subgroup; and asylum seekers may be particularly wary of authority figures seeking information, given their precarious residency status. Access by researchers in Australia to detention centres remains an insurmountable challenge, with government authorities failing to endorse studies by independent investigators. In spite of these challenges, a number of studies have been completed with substantial convergence in results. In the UK Bracken and Gorst-Unsworth (1991) documented evidence of torture in six of the ten cases of detained asylum seekers they treated. All ten suffered from major depression and four were suicidal, with two having made suicide attempts. In another UK-based study, Pourgerides and colleagues (1995) found that the majority of detained asylum seekers (n=15) gave histories of traumatic experience prior to exile, including exposure to systematic torture. As in the study by Bracken and Gorst-Unsworth, the most common psychiatric problems were depression and post-traumatic stress symptoms. Profound despair and suicidal ideation, including an attempted hanging, were recorded. The asylum seekers expressed 'a profound sense of injustice (in relation to) their reception and treatment…detention is seen as punitive, hostile and unfair' (p. 96).

Table 5.1 Post-migration stresses and health access difficulties faced by asylum seekers (percentages)

	Fears of %	Forced %	Extreme stresses Worries %	Obstacle %	Poverty %	Emergency %	Severe access difficulties Long-term %	Dental %	Counselling %
Asylum Seekers Study (Sydney)	81	42	39	50	33	52	49	67	
Tamil Community Study (Sydney)	68	63	71	30	18	60	69	63	34
East Timorese Study (Sydney)	85	85	89	70	70	48	52	52	96

Table 5.2 Human rights abuses and trauma experienced by asylum seekers

	N	Origin %	Sample %	Exposed to murder or killing %	Life threat %	Forced isolation/ separation %	Harassed, injured, assaulted %	Sexually abused %	Tortured %	Combat exposure %	Political imprisonment %	Ill-health, no medical care %
Asylum Seekers Centre Study (Sydney)	40	21 countries	Consecutive attenders at English class	58	44	42	32		26			32
Tamil Survey (Sydney)	62	Sri Lanka	Snowball Community Survey	39	40	27	13	0	26	23	19	40
East Timorese Study (Victoria)	50	East Timor	Clients of torture/ trauma service, 17 in detention	60		46	84		68		56	
East Timorese Study (Sydney)	33	East Timor	Outreach service	83	61	70	57	26	43	57	43	83
Maribyrnong Detention Centre (Victoria)	25	Sri Lanka	Detention	92	88	84		24	72	40		

Tables 5.1 and 5.2 summarise studies undertaken in Australia both in the community and in detention. Although diverse in methodologies and sampling methods, some studies managed to access almost entire cohorts of asylum seeker populations at a given point in time. For example, the study undertaken at the Maribyrnong Detention Centre (Thompson et al. 1998) involved almost all the Tamils detained there at that time and many of the cohorts were followed up by the researchers after release, allowing clinical verification of findings over time. Similarly, the participant observer study at Villawood Detention Centre in Sydney (Sultan & O'Sullivan 2001) involved thirty-three of thirty-seven detainees held for longer than six months, and the detained doctor who undertook the study was directly familiar with the longitudinal course of each subject.

Levels of trauma exposure across all studies were high (table 5.1) but varied according to ethnic grouping and background as would be predicted. For example, across studies, direct exposure to murder varied between 27 per cent and 92 per cent; to personal life threat, between 44 per cent and 88 per cent; and to torture, 26 per cent to 72 per cent. In the studies that assessed this variable, ill-health without access to medical care in the country of origin varied between 32 per cent and 83 per cent. Overall, levels of trauma reported were consistent in magnitude, type and range with those found among authorised refugees worldwide, suggesting that asylum seekers form an integral subgroup of the larger population of persons with legitimate claims to protection.

Rates of PTSD, depression, and anxiety in these samples were uniformly high. In the Sydney asylum seekers centre study (Silove et al. 1997) which included a wide range of ethnic groups, 33 per cent exceeded threshold scores for depression and 23 per cent for anxiety on the Hopkins symptom checklist. Thirty-eight per cent met criteria for PTSD. In the Sydney study of Tamils living in the community (Silove et al. 1998), symptoms of anxiety, depression, and PTSD in asylum seekers were similar to those in refugees and exceeded levels in compatriot immigrants by an order of three to four.

Asylum seekers in detention appear to be unusually symptomatic. The detained group of Tamils at Maribyrnong Detention Centre in Victoria (Thompson et al. 1998) returned much higher scores on all indices—suicidality, panic, depression, PTSD, somatic distress, and anxiety—compared to compatriot asylum seekers living in the community. These findings are supported by the Villawood study (Sultan & O'Sullivan 2001) in which all but one of the 33 participants were judged on clinical grounds to have had a psychiatric disturbance at some point during detention. Sixty-five per cent reported pronounced suicidal urges, and 57 per cent had been prescribed psychotropic medications, mainly antidepressants. Behavioural disturbances among detainees were common, including psychotic reactions, extreme rage, profound withdrawal, and extensive somatic complaints. The qualitative aspect of this study was of great importance in that the doctor and psychologist responsible for the report were able to observe first-hand the progressive deterioration in levels of depression over time, with exacerbations being heralded by successive milestones in the administrative assessment process.

Studies among asylum seekers in the community have revealed high levels of stress associated with post-migration stressors, many imposed by the administrative policies imposed on this group (Steel et al. 1999). Separation from family, poverty and unemployment, difficulties accessing health and counselling services, boredom and isolation, fears of repatriation, and the complexity of administrative procedures all figure high on the list of stresses identified by asylum seekers in Australia (Sinnerbrink et al. 1996). The post-migration stresses appear to exert a largely independent impact on post-traumatic stress symptoms, thereby adding to the effects of pre-migration trauma (Steel et al. 1999). Instead of gradual stabilisation and adaptation, the expected trajectory for most refugees once they reach a place of safety, asylum seekers appear to show a pattern of progressive worsening in psychological functioning, a course that seems substantially attributable to the restrictions imposed on this group.

Villains or victims?

As indicated above, statements made by political leaders in Australia often highlight the extreme reactions of asylum seekers, particularly those in detention, in an effort to depict their behaviours as manipulative, unscrupulous, or as posing a threat to security. Hence, detainees are held primarily responsible for acts of violence and confrontation, for embarking on hunger strikes, for self-damaging behaviour and for escape attempts. In early 2002, two hundred asylum seekers including adolescents, embarked on a hunger strike at Woomera, one of the most remote detention centres located in a semi-desert environment in South Australia. During the ensuing controversy, claims were made that adults had sewn the lips of children together to prevent them from eating. The inference drawn by political leaders is that the host society is justified in rejecting persons with alien cultural behaviours since the newcomers would not integrate into society. It seems more likely that the disturbed behaviours manifested are an outcome of a self-fulfilling prophecy in which the conditions in detention provoke and encourage uncharacteristically desperate behaviours. In Australia, new detention centres have been located in remote regions, thousands of kilometres from the nearest major city. In all these centres, access to a full range of legal, social and health services is limited, as is contact with compatriot communities and relatives settled in the larger metropolitan areas. The Human Rights and Equal Opportunity Commission (1999) has suggested that the boredom and frustration of prolonged detention together with social isolation may be responsible for outbreaks of violence, including domestic violence, among detainees and between detainees and officials. Claims have been made of the use of solitary confinement and other punitive measures to quell dissent, with detainees living in a state of intimidation and passivity, often for prolonged periods of time (Silove & Kinzie 2001).

Asylum seekers feel trapped in a continuum of anxiety and fear in which there is a convergence of experiences from the past, the present and the future that makes effective adaptive responses increasingly difficult. Memories of past dangers and humiliations intermingle with current insecurities and frustrations, feelings that, in turn, are magnified by fears of future persecution should detainees be involuntarily repatriated. Recollections of past imprisonment merge with recurrent feelings of outrage at being confined behind razor wire in the country in which the asylum seeker has sought freedom. The sense of loss of control over one's personal life, a pervasive and inescapable reality when living under repressive regimes, is further provoked by the uncompromising regime of control experienced in the detention centre. The future is perceived as resting entirely in the hands of an incomprehensible bureaucratic machinery that is experienced as alien and impersonal, hence intensifying past feelings of helplessness in the face of an arbitrary and unjust system of authority.

The intensive administrative inquiry applied to test refugee claims can provoke heightened anxiety, and in those previously subjected to interrogation, torture, and other forms of extreme abuse, dissociative reactions can occur. During the inquiry, memories can become incoherent and fragmented thereby interfering with the capacity of applicants to provide a consistent and consecutive account of their histories. Yet inaccuracies and inconsistencies in testimony are often cited as the primary reason for dismissing refugee claims (Christianson & Safer 1996; Deng 2000; Summerfield 1995). Tragically, the long arm of torture can reach far beyond the torture chamber and interfere with the capacity of survivors to achieve protection from further persecution.

Reactions of rage, paranoia, extreme social withdrawal, passivity, and acts of desperation such as violence, hunger strikes and escapes, may all reflect the progressive exhaustion of survival strategies that have been tested and undermined through a succession of hostile obstacles in the country of origin, during the period of flight, and finally, in the country where the asylum seeker invested all remaining hopes of gaining refuge.

The key element that can modulate the pervasive sense of threat is the enduring faith that a benevolent protector will intercede—in this instance—the trust is invested in Australia's reputation as a humane society. As indicated earlier, what made the Refugee Convention such a landmark in humanitarian law was precisely the centrality it gave to this principle; that somewhere in the world, persons fleeing persecution could be assured of finding refuge. When faith in that international promise is eroded, particularly for those in long-term detention, extreme forms of psychological disintegration can occur. Although at one level, it may be accurate to diagnose such persons as suffering from a profound depression (Sultan & O'Sullivan 2001), a deeper understanding of the underlying forces at play is also necessary; recognition that the desperate reactions that are manifested reflect a final capitulation to hopelessness when detainees at last realise that the quest for security and a life with dignity is unrealisable.

Discussion

The pitfalls of Australia's recent attempt to implement an idiosyncratic local solution to the problem of asylum underscores the importance of understanding the historical and contemporary context of displacement at a global level. When such universal issues are ignored, policy contradictions emerge and actions that may be well-intentioned can have destructive impacts.

Forced displacement is a fact of history that is unlikely to disappear in the foreseeable future. One of the surest outcomes of war, mass conflict, and oppression is the flow of displaced persons across national borders— seeking protection for oneself and one's family is a natural impetus driven by deeply ingrained evolutionary mechanisms. Without considering the root causes of such population flows, leaders of recipient countries whose sole concern is to stem the influx are likely to employ methods of deterrence that increasingly resemble the arbitrary and unjust experiences from which displaced persons are fleeing in the first instance. Australia is coming close to falling into this trap. In particular, regimes that use torture and other forms of oppression inevitably justify their actions by public propaganda that vilifies the victims and blames them for their plight, usually by accusing them of representing a threat to the integrity and sovereignty of the state. It is ironic that recipient countries such as Australia are resorting to the same claims to justify the rejection of asylum seekers.

To think clearly about global strategies in dealing with the challenge of asylum, some key principles need to be highlighted. Asylum seekers in Western countries represent only one small component of the much larger and heterogeneous group of displaced persons worldwide. The majority of this larger population comprise groups displaced within their own countries or who have fled to neighbouring states, most commonly underdeveloped countries of Africa, Asia, and the Middle East. Hence, even with the increase in flow of asylum seekers in the last decade, the responsibility for care and resettlement falls mainly on the underdeveloped, not the developed countries.

Hence, in considering asylum policy, countries of the West need to reappraise what the full meaning of being a developed country is. There is an increasing tendency to equate development with material wealth—if so, the rejection of asylum seekers represents a brazen act of selfishness—excluding the poor from a share in the riches. The deliberate confusion in public terminology used in which asylum seekers frequently are referred to as illegal or unauthorised economic migrants, suggests that such narrow motives may be exerting a powerful influence in determining asylum policies. Leaders of the West, in their support for globalisation, reveal their true motives by extolling the virtues of free trade while at the same time erecting greater barriers to the free movement of people. The self-interest motive is buttressed by appeals to other primitive mechanisms such as territoriality, latent racism, and to raw forms of nationalism. The arrival of unheralded and unauthorised asylum seekers can easily be represented as an invasion, an affront to the rights of countries to control their borders, and a threat to the cultural integrity of the society.

Leaders can choose to use the easy target of asylum seekers to polarise the society whenever this appears to be politically advantageous. On deeper reflection, they might recognise that this stratagem actually poses a threat to the notion of development both in relation to the host country and the asylum group. Adherence to the mission of development has a double-edge since the advantages it confers are matched by a set of obligations. A developed society is one in which civil rights are defended even if there are costs involved in ensuring the psychosocial well-being of all sectors of the population without discrimination, and in maintaining a commitment to building human capacities in a manner that offers opportunities for the advancement of all persons. Globalisation means many things but one core element is the extension of the notion of development beyond national borders and the constraints of individual citizenship. Development thus represents a vision of society in which administration is transparent, in which justice, participation and respect for democratic processes are extended to all, and in which the building of human capacities and opportunities is given priority. The focus on capacity building and the enhancement of opportunities without artificial restrictions represents a point of growing consensus and convergence in the human sciences, in fields as diverse as the human rights movement, development economics, and mental health promotion and prevention. It is noteworthy that humanitarian relief and development initiatives undertaken by Western countries in post-conflict societies such as East Timor, Kosovo, and Afghanistan are underpinned by these principles, indicating a commitment to the universality of this world vision of development.

The treatment of asylum seekers in Australia, and, to a variable degree in other developed countries, thus represents a contradiction within a world order ostensibly committed to development. Suspending the development of a subgroup by restricting the capacity of its members to participate meaningfully in society is antithetical to this notion. The contradiction becomes ever more stark where members of the very same community are treated diametrically differently simply by virtue of their geographical location and their administrative status. So, for example, East Timorese exiles who fled to Australia were forced to live under conditions of restriction and deprivation for years. They faced unemployment, poverty, isolation, and difficulties associated with accessing services. Since 1999 the Australian Government has made major contributions to developing aid programs in the emerging nation of East Timor. The distinction, in response, once again, is based entirely on the salience given to crossing national borders. Ultimately, then, thinking on this issue appears to be caught at the crossroads between the rhetoric of globalisation and the limited self-interest associated with narrow notions of nationalism and national self-interest. Asylum seekers are the group trapped at the crossroads between these age-old fortress mentalities and a vision of a just world order. As individuals, they are enduring a great deal of suffering as a consequence.

Recommended reading

Jupp, J. (2002) *From White Australia to Woomera: the story of Australian Immigration*, Cambridge University Press, Cambridge.

McMaster, D. (2001) *Asylum seekers. Australia's response to refugees*, Melbourne University Press, Melbourne.

Silove, D. & Steel, Z. (2002) Matters Arising: Asylum seekers and healthcare, *Medical Journal of Australia*, 176: 86.

Sinnerbrink, I., Silove, D., Manicavasagar, V., Steel, Z. & Field, A. (1996) Asylum seekers: general health status and problems with access to health care, *Medical Journal of Australia*, 165: 634–7.

Steel, Z. & Silove, D. (2001) The mental health implications of detaining asylum seekers, *Medical Journal of Australia*, 175: 596–9.

Sultan, A. & O'Sullivan, K. (2001) Psychological disturbances in asylum seekers held in long term detention: a participant–observer account, *Medical Journal of Australia*, 175: 593–6.

UNHCR (2001) Guidelines on the Detention of Asylum Seekers, In Gee, A. (ed) *Pre-reading materials for 'Misunderstanding asylum seekers'* A Symposium on Truth, Myth and Justice in Australia, pp. 19–27.

References

Bracken, P. & Gorst-Unsworth, C. (1991) The mental state of detained asylum seekers, *Psychiatry Bulletin*, 15: 657–9.

Christianson, S. & Safer, M. (1996) Emotional events and emotions in autobiographical memories, In Rubin, D. (ed) *Remembering our past: studies in autobiographical memory*, Cambridge University Press, Cambridge, pp. 218–41.

de Jong, J., Komproe, I., Van Ommeren, M., El Masri, M., Araya, M., Khaled, N., van De Put, W. & Somasundaram, D. (2001) Lifetime events and posttraumatic stress disorder in 4 postconflict settings, *Journal of the American Medical Association*, 286(5): 555–62.

Deng, F. (2000) Conclusion: The cause of justice behind civil wars, In Amadiume, I. & An-Na'im, A. (eds) *The politics of memory. Truth, healing and social justice*, Zed Books, London, pp. 184–200.

Grant, B. (1979) *The Boat People: An 'Age' Investigation with Bruce Grant*, Penguin, Ringwood.

Human Rights and Equal Opportunity Commission (1999) 1998–99 Review of immigration detention centres, In vol. 2001 HREOC, Canberra. Available at: http://www.hreoc.gov.au/pdf/human_rights/asylum_seekers/idc_review.pdf.

Mollica, R., Donelan, K., Tor, S., Lavelle, J., Elias, C., Frankel, M. & Blendon, R. (1993) The effect of trauma and confinement on functional health and mental health status of Cambodians living in Thailand–Cambodia border camps, *Journal of the American Medical Association*, 270: 581–6.

Mollica, R., Wyshak, G., de Marneffe, D. & et al. (1987) Indochinese versions of the Hopkins Symptom Checklist 25: A screening instrument for the psychiatric care of refugees, *American Journal of Psychiatry*, 144: 497–500.

Pourgourides, C., Sashidharan, S. & Braken, P. (1995) *A Second Exile: the mental health implications of detention of asylum seekers in the United Kingdom*, North Birmingham Mental Health NHS Trust, Birmingham.

Shrestha, N., Sharma, B., van Ommeren, M., Regmi, S., Makaju, R., Kamproe, I., Sheshtha, G. & de Jong, J. (1998) Impact of torture on refugees displaced within the developing world, *Journal of the American Medical Association*, 280: 443–8.

Silove, D. & Ekblad, S. (1998) Proposals for the Development of Mental Health and Psychosocial Services in Refugee Camps: 18 August, (ed) Consultant Report to the United Nations High Commissioner for Refugees, pp. 1–52.

Silove, D. & Kinzie, J.D. (2001) Survivors of war trauma, mass violence, and civilian terror, In Gerrity, E., Keane, T.M. & Tuma, F. (eds), *The mental health consequences of torture*, Kluwer Academic/Plenum Publishers, Inc., New York, pp. 159–74.

Silove, D., McIntosh, P. & Becker, R. (1993) Risk of retraumatisation of asylum-seekers in Australia, *Australian & New Zealand Journal of Psychiatry*, 27(5): 606–12.

Silove, D., Sinnerbrink, I., Field, A., Manicavasagar, V. & Steel, Z. (1997) Anxiety, depression and PTSD in asylum seekers: associations with pre-migration trauma and post-migration stressors, *British Journal of Psychiatry*, 170: 351–7.

Silove, D., Steel, Z., McGorry, P. & Mohan, P. (1998) Trauma exposure, postmigration stressors, and symptoms of anxiety, depression and posttraumatic stress in Tamil asylum seekers: comparisons with refugees and immigrants, *Acta Psychiatrica Scandinavica*, 97(3): 175–81.

Sinnerbrink, I., Silove, D., Manicavasagar, V., Steel, Z. & Field, A. (1996) Asylum seekers: general health status and problems with access to health care, *Medical Journal of Australia*, 165: 634–7.

Steel, Z. & Silove, D. (2001) The mental health implications of detaining asylum seekers, *Medical Journal of Australia*, 175: 596–9.

Steel, Z., Silove, D., Bird, K., McGorry, P. & Mohan, P. (1999) Pathways from War Trauma to Posttraumatic Stress Symptoms Among Tamil Asylum Seekers, Refugees, and Immigrants, *Journal of Traumatic Stress*, 12(3): 421–35.

Sultan, A. & O'Sullivan, K. (2001) Psychological disturbances in asylum seekers held in long term detention: a participant–observer account, *Medical Journal of Australia*, 175: 593–6.

Summerfield, D. (1995) Raising the dead: war, reparation, and the politics of memory, *British Medical Journal*, 311(7003): 495–7.

Thompson, M., McGorry, P., Silove, D. & Steel, Z. (1998) Maribyrnong Detention Centre Tamil Survey *The mental health and well-being of on shore asylum seekers in Australia*, The Psychiatry Research & Teaching Unit, Sydney, pp. 27–31.

Van Ommeren, M., de Jong Joop, T., Sharma, B. et al.(2001) Psychiatric disorders among tortured Bhutanese refugees in Nepal, *Archives of General Psychiatry*, 58: 475–82.

6

Double Jeopardy: Children Seeking Asylum

Eileen Pittaway and Linda Bartolomei

Introduction

Australia is the only country in the developed world which places refugee and asylum seeking children into mandatory and arbitrary detention while the individual or family claim for asylum is assessed (Refugee Council of Australia 2002). This is contrary to our obligations to a number of Human Rights Conventions, which the Australian Government has both signed and ratified. The most important of these is the Convention on the Rights of the Child (CRC).

The changing nature of war and warfare in the latter part of the twentieth century has meant that now, more than ever before, civilians are the focus of battles, armed conflict, and torture. This exposes more people, including children, to trauma, with devastating consequences (Goldson 1996). It has generated an unprecedented global movement of peoples, as large populations are forced from their countries and their homes by armed conflict and fear of persecution. Since 1975 the number of refugees in the world has swelled from an estimated 11 million to 20 million in 2002, with an additional 20 to 25 million internally displaced peoples. UNHCR estimates that 50 per cent of these refugee and displaced people are children under the age of 18 (UNHCR 2002).

It is estimated that of the approximately 12,000 people who migrate to Australia annually as part of the Refugee and Special Humanitarian Intake about 40 per cent are children and young people. Many of these children have suffered from severe hardship, they have had their sense of safety violated, suffered physical abuse, neglect, abandonment, sexual abuse and exploitation, some have been forced to fight as child soldiers and most have witnessed torture and/or been tortured themselves. They have watched fathers, brothers, and uncles being killed, or have seen them 'disappear'. Many watched as their mothers, sisters, aunts were tortured and raped (UNHCR 1994).

Increasing numbers of these children are unaccompanied minors, children not accompanied by a custodial adult, claiming asylum in their own right. Minors are defined in international law as people below 18 years of age. There are several circumstances that can result in unaccompanied minors, including families sending their children away to seek asylum to escape conscription as child soldiers. Other reasons are to escape targeting by authorities, punishment for political activity, or to seek a place of safety for a family in danger. Some of those reaching Australia are as young as 12 years old.

The groundwork for the protection of children was laid in the first Declaration of the Rights of the Child in 1924. Since then, international child protection has slowly evolved through statements on the special care and protection to which motherhood and childhood are entitled in the 1948 Universal Declaration of Human Rights to the adoption of the CRC 1989 (United Nations 1989). All but two of the countries (Somalia and the United States of America) that are members of the United Nations have ratified the CRC making it the most universally ratified treaty to date. The CRC remains a dynamic document with the recent addition of two protocols that deal with contemporary issues affecting children, namely children's involvement in armed conflict and child trafficking in the sex industry.

The intention of this convention, which is legally binding on state parties, is to obtain an unequivocal declaration and acceptance of the obligation of all humans to protect and ensure the best interests of the child. Of particular relevance to the topic of this volume is the acknowledgment of the challenge of meeting this obligation in the context of conflict, displacement, and resettlement of children. Article 22 states:

> **1** States Parties shall take appropriate measures to ensure that a child who is seeking refugee status or who is considered a refugee in accordance with applicable international or domestic law and procedures shall whether unaccompanied or accompanied by his or her parents or by any other person receive appropriate protection and humanitarian assistance in the enjoyment of applicable rights set forth in the present convention and in other international human rights or humanitarian instruments to which the said States are Parties
>
> **2** … in cases where no parents or other members of the family can be found, the child shall be accorded the same protection as any other child permanently or temporarily deprived of his or her family environment for any reason.

This chapter highlights the arguments of possible violations of children's rights within the context of detention in a country of asylum, in this case, Australia and the impact of this on the children and their families. While some of the issues discussed are also covered in other human rights conventions (see Kneebone and Allotey p. 1), the main focus in this chapter is on the CRC.

Australia's response to child asylum seekers

Australia currently mandates the detention of asylum seekers, including children and unaccompanied minors as a critical component of the policy of deterrence designed to combat 'people smuggling' (Crock 1993). Management of the detention centres is outsourced to a private firm. Those who are detained remain in detention until their claims for asylum have been assessed. Those who are recognised as refugees are granted a protection visa but remain in detention until their health and character checks have been completed. This process may take anything from a matter of weeks to several years.

The right to seek and enjoy protection from persecution is a fundamental right enshrined in the Universal Declaration of Human Rights (Article 14) (United Nations Department of Public Information). The responsibilities of countries to provide protection are set out in the 1951 Convention Relating to the Status of Refugees. In addition to this obligation, signatory states are obliged to honour their commitments to international human rights standards. These include commitments to ensure the human rights of asylum seekers within their borders are not violated while asylum claims are processed. These rights are addressed in a number of conventions including the International Convention on Civil and Political Rights (ICCPR), the Convention on the Elimination of all forms of Discrimination Against Women (CEDAW) and the Convention on the Rights of the Child (CRC). Australia has signed and ratified these conventions, although only the commitments made under the CRC have been substantially incorporated into Australian domestic law.

The mandatory detention policy has raised some protest in the community because of the apparent violation of a number of articles in the CRC, including:

> States Parties shall take all appropriate measures to ensure that the child is protected against all forms of discrimination or punishment on the basis of status, activities, expressed opinions or beliefs of the child's parents, legal guardians, or family members

Article 2 (2)

States Parties recognize the right of every child to a standard of living adequate for the child's physical, mental, spiritual, moral and social development ...

Article 27 (1)

States Parties shall ensure that no child shall be deprived of his or her liberty unlawfully or arbitrarily. The arrest, detention or imprisonment of a child shall be in conformity with the law and shall be used only as a measure of last resort and for the shortest appropriate period of time.

Article 37 (2b)

Every child deprived of his or her liberty shall have the right to prompt access to legal and other appropriate assistance, as well as the right to challenge the legality of the *deprivation of his or her liberty before a court or other competent, independent and impartial authority and to a prompt decision on any such action.*

Article 37 (2d)
(emphasis added)

Preliminary research into the effects of detention on refugee children was conducted by the Australian National Committee on Refugee Women (ANCORW) and the Centre for Refugee Research UNSW (CRR) in 2000 (Pittaway & Maksimovic 2000). The research design was restricted by the ability to obtain a broad and representative range of participants because access to detention centres is restricted and tightly controlled. People working in the centres, including full-time staff and visiting personnel, such as lawyers and psychologists and even volunteers, are bound by confidentiality agreements with the detention centre management. In addition, most asylum seekers found to have valid claims for asylum and released into the community on three-year Temporary Protection Visas are generally reticent about describing conditions in the centres because they believe that if they do, the government will revoke their visas. The findings reported are therefore based on data combining a comprehensive review of the relevant international literature with in-depth case study interviews conducted with some key service providers, visitors, and a limited number of current and former detainees who accepted our guarantee of anonymity.

The experience and effects of detention on children

Asylum seekers by definition often claim to have undergone torture, trauma, or some other form of persecution within their own country.

Many have also suffered horrific experiences during their escape to a country of asylum (Pittaway & Breen 1999). UNHCR estimates that the majority of all refugee women and many children are routinely raped and sexually abused (UNHCR 1995). Many children are born to refugee women as the result of rape, many of whom are subsequently rejected by their families (Forbes Martin 1991). It is evident that refugee children are extremely vulnerable (Ajdukovic 1993; Allodi 1980a, b; Athey & Ahearn 1991; Garbarino et al. 1991; UNHCR 1994) and need intensive support to enable them to address and deal with pre-arrival experiences. Children seeking asylum, whether with other family members or unaccompanied would necessarily include those who have undergone the persecution that qualifies them as refugees and have also faced the stresses of the journey to Australia. Detention of indefinite duration can only add to the trauma of these children. Child detainees live behind razor wire, surrounded by uniforms, identification badges, roll calls and searches (Rayner 2001).

A major concern identified in the literature review and confirmed by several of the key service providers were the negative mental health effects on individuals of living in a confined 'community' in an atmosphere of unrelieved tension and stress, where there is a large mix of cultures, ages, and sexes. Visitors to Australia's detention centres reported harrowing stories of the conditions in which asylum seekers, including children, were detained. These included the use of solitary confinement to punish children for minor misdemeanours, such as being cheeky to guards; of the incessant screaming of disturbed and distressed detainees; of the constant noise of loud speaker announcements; of the vacant empty expressions of the children; and of personal accounts of violence and sexual abuse (Pittaway & Bartolomei 2001).

The negative impacts of detention are further exacerbated by a lack of appropriate facilities and poorly trained staff who are frequently insensitive, unsympathetic or aggressive. A child of eight years witnessed '... the forcible rounding up, the handcuffing and removal of a small party of her co-nationals ... It took place in her classroom to which she refuses to return lest it happen there again, but this time to her and her loved ones' (Molony 2000).

Detainees, including children, reported difficulty in sleeping and eating. Many reported experiencing regular nightmares. This combined with routine awakening by guards using flashlights during random night patrols, led to reports of fear associated with sleep. The practice of mixing different ethnic groups within the same sleeping quarters led to some detainees fearing harassment or injury from members of those ethnic groups that persecuted them in their countries of origin, and also contributed to insomnia (Rogalla & Highfield 2001).

The experience of detention is heavily influenced by the behaviour of other detainees who form a major part of children's daily lives. In 1998 the Australian Human Rights and Equal Opportunity Commission (HREOC) conducted an inquiry into Australia's treatment of asylum seekers. The findings suggested that the boredom and frustration of prolonged detention was responsible for outbreaks of violence, including domestic violence, among detainees and officials. Of particular concern is the exposure of children to suicide attempts and other forms of self-harm by other detainees.

> I spent nearly four years in Australian detention. Two women tried to commit suicide. There are no words to describe what it is really like in there. I spent four years without real schooling and without social life… I couldn't believe that this was Australia. Now that I've got to know Australians, I realise they are not like the government. A lot of them do not know what the Australian government does to people… I'm twenty-one and still doing the HSC.
>
> (Vinson & Lester 1998)

HREOC commenced a National Inquiry into Children in Immigration Detention in Australia, in early 2002. In addition to receiving submissions from service providers, lawyers, and advocacy groups the inquiry received submissions from a broad range of professionals who had been employed in immigration detention centres. These included psychologists, medical practitioners, nurses, and teachers. Testimony provided to the inquiry by the majority of these professionals confirms that children in detention centres continue to regularly witness suicide attempts and incidents of self-harm by other detainees.

> There was very visible self harm, constant talk of it. The children for example when I arrived would have seen people in graves—when I first arrived there were people in dug graves with children seeing this. Some of the children—it was their parents or people they knew. They knew why the parents were doing this. They knew that the parents were talking about possibly dying. They were on a hunger strike. There was visible self harming on the razor wire. People were taken to the medical centre at regular intervals having slashed themselves. There were attempted hangings that these children would have seen.
>
> (Bender 2002)

A HREOC report also highlighted the concern that single women and unaccompanied minors were at increased risk of abuse and exploitation when confined in mixed-sex detention facilities (Human Rights and Equal Opportunity Commission 1999). Further attention has been drawn to this concern by allegations of sexual abuse of children in detention.

> I have no doubt in my mind that child sex abuse has happened. And I think that if we look at the environment that has been established there, where you are putting people of different ethnic backgrounds, you're putting people who might be criminals or those genuinely seeking asylum here in our country, and you put children into that mix as well, then the imbalance of power means that there's going to be abuses occurring.
>
> (West 2000)

> ... there were a worrying number of reports of indecent assault and threats toward unattached women and children who represent the groups at highest risk. In my view, the accommodation and monitoring/care arrangements at Immigration Detention Centres did not come up to what I would regard as a minimum acceptable standard to ensure that those at greatest risk are not exposed to harm.
>
> (Commonwealth Ombudsman 2001)

There have also been allegations of centre management (ACM) ordering the suppression of reports of suspected child sexual abuse. This was substantiated by a parliamentary inquiry (Flood 2001). A number of submissions provided to the HREOC Inquiry into Children in Immigration Detention raise concerns regarding the lack of appropriate policies and procedures for addressing allegations of child abuse, including sexual abuse (Bender 2002; Huxstep 2002). While many of these issues may be the direct responsibility of the private firm that has been contracted to manage the centre, the government is ultimately responsible to ensure the protection of human rights within the institution. This is addressed within the CRC.

> States Parties shall ensure that the institutions, services and facilities responsible for the care or protection of children shall conform with the standards established by competent authorities, particularly in the areas of safety, health, in the number and suitability of their staff, as well as competent supervision.
>
> Article 3 (3)

Recreation and education

The rights of ALL children, in whichever country they currently reside and regardless of their legal status are clearly articulated in CRC. These rights do not just cover basic needs such as food and shelter. They also include the right to health care, to education, to recreation and leisure. Human rights instruments stress our obligations to respect the dignity of all people. Important articles of CRC that are clearly contravened by the detention of asylum seekers, especially children, include:

> The development of respect for human rights and fundamental freedoms, and for the principles enshrined in the Charter of the United Nations ...
>
> Article 28 (1b)

> The preparation of the child for responsible life in a free society, in the spirit of understanding, peace, tolerance, equality of sexes, and friendship among all peoples, ethnic, national and religious groups and persons of indigenous origin
>
> Article 28 (1d)

> States Parties shall agree that the education of the child be directed to:
> The development of the child's personality, talents and mental and physical abilities to their fullest potential
>
> Article 29 (1a)

> States Parties recognize the right of the child to rest and leisure, to engage in play and recreational activities appropriate to the age of the child and to participate freely in cultural life and the arts
>
> Article 31 (1)

The conditions in Australian detention centres demonstrate the extent of the challenge of meeting the above obligations under the circumstances. The findings of the CRR research and the HREOC inquiry indicate that the conditions, resources, and teaching standards within detention centres are inadequate to meet the educational needs of the children.

Very often, the education system within detention centres does not promote an environment of positive learning experiences or activities for students. Rather, for many it is an environment that promotes fear and apprehension. It is a general requirement that for children's learning to be facilitated they must be provided with continuity and quality in teaching. Schooling for children in detention is provided on an ad hoc basis. The use of part-time teaching staff, a lack of consistent standards of teaching and different levels of teacher expertise mean that this does not happen in Australia's detention centres. The age groups vary within the class depending on the incoming and outgoing numbers of asylum seekers and none of the children receive full-time schooling.

Unlike the legislated system in Australian schools, the teaching curriculum within the detention centres is left to the discretion of the teacher(s). This results in lack of coordination and continuity of the curriculum and confusion for the children. In addition, in some detention centres, non-academic programs for children are being introduced by community groups, without coordination with the education staff. Despite the efforts of committed teachers, the education offered to children within detention centres not only falls below the standard of Australian schools, but also lacks quality in its content and style of delivery.

The importance of restoring some level of cultural normalcy in the lives of refugee children cannot be overemphasised. Informal educational opportunities for play and exploration play a critical role in re-establishing normal community life and in positive child development (Andrews & Ben-Arieh 1999; UNHCR 1992). Play is essential to children's physical, social, and cognitive development (UNHCR 1994 pp. 38–9). Recreation facilities vary across the detention centres. Children incarcerated in the Port Headland detention centre have no play facilities, they share what recreational space there is with the adults and have access to the ball ground only between 2pm and 2.30pm, which is the hottest time of the day. In Villawood and Maribyrnong Detention Centres in Sydney and Melbourne, a program of excursions for some of the detained children has been recently instigated. This is not available to all children as some are considered likely to abscond. Volunteers report that while there is no doubt the children do enjoy the excursions and getting out of the detention centre, due to the lack of teachers, time, and resources on their return to Villawood, there is no opportunity for the children to reflect on this positive experience through drawings or discussions during school. In addition, in order to avoid conflict and jealousy, the children who are allowed on the excursions keep quiet about their experiences. This fear of telling what they have done has an ongoing impact for the children's social development in forming relationships (Pittaway & Bartolomei 2001).

Opportunities for children to socialise with peers and the benefits from having an intimate friend of their own age with whom to share their ideas and experiences are as important as formal education. Feeling accepted by the peer group and being able to share school experiences and intimate confidences with one or more close friends are crucial to happiness in middle childhood and helps shape the child's social development (Peterson 1996 p. 260).

The small number of children within detention at any one time and the variation in the age, culture, and language groups often inhibits children from forming social relationships with children of a similar age. They often become suspicious of people who are not fellow detainees and become distant with those who try to work with them. This, combined with the lack of recreational space for children in detention centres, often results in the children associating with young adults. Consequently, children as young as 12 take an active role in political activities, such as hunger strikes and sewing their lips together. Food assumes a major role in asserting control within a powerless situation and nutrition becomes a major issue. Apart from the psychological effects this might have, childhood malnutrition inhibits mental and physical development and increases vulnerability to infections (UNHCR 1994 p. 58). It is not uncommon for refugees and asylum seekers in general, but children in particular to have a poor nutritional status on arrival which can be further exacerbated. It is of great concern that three of the service providers interviewed indicated that children within detention react to the stressful conditions by refusing to eat or being unable to hold their food down.

In the longer term, when these children get out of detention and begin the process of integration into schools within the community, they experience severe difficulties in their learning. These partly result from the breaks in education due to their flight from their homelands, but are contributed to by the piece-meal pattern and low standard of education they have received during the detention period (Pittaway & Breen 1999; Pittaway & Maksimovic 2000).

Health effects

A recent research report by Silove, Steel and Watter (2000) states that the 'potentially deleterious effect of detention on the mental health of asylum seekers has been raised repeatedly' (p. 608). They identify indicators of this, which include high rates of attempted suicide and hunger strikes. They cite a study by Thompson et al. (1988) conducted with 25 detained Tamils, which found that they displayed twice the level of war related trauma when compared with compatriot asylum seekers and refugees living in the community. While they urge constraint in drawing definitive conclusions from these studies, given the difficulties in accessing facilities and sampling, there is a convergence with the interview data provided by human rights groups and involved health professionals which indicates that detention is a powerful contributor to psychological distress in asylum seekers.

Features that emerge across studies on the psychological and psychosocial effects of incarceration in Australian detention centres suggest that both adults and children present as depressed and anxious. Their responses to events and circumstances are characterised by sadness, lack of energy, and disinterest. They are frightened for their personal safety and worried about their families back home (Crock 1993 p. 85). More recent work undertaken by Steele and Sultan (2001) provides further evidence of the degree to which detention compounds refugee trauma.

The traumas experienced by refugee children can cause a range of symptoms including anger, hostility, nightmares, and severe dysfunctional behaviour, and delayed development. If they are not addressed, the results are long lasting and debilitating and are often compounded by the unwillingness of refugees from some ethnic backgrounds to seek or accept treatment for what they regard as mental illness (Pittaway 1998). The attached stigma breeds shame and humiliation.

One psychological factor unique to children is that they are still developing. Their personalities are being formed and social and coping skills are being learnt on a daily basis. The children in detention are socially and culturally isolated. Instead of fostering positive development, the experience of detention is more likely to produce antisocial and aggressive behaviour. Many children who are detained undergo behavioural changes caused by the stressful living conditions in the detention centre, and their unknown future. Such changes may include loss of appetite, insomnia, crying, withdrawal, and increased dependency. The child may, in addition, sense the tension and stress its parents feel as a result of the parents' uncertainty about the future, boredom, and lack of support in caring for their children while in detention. These combined factors lead to delayed and dysfunctional psychosocial and emotional development in the children.

The HREOC investigation into the prolonged effects of children in detention on children documented this statement from a young Cambodian unattached minor who was in detention for five years.

In the last year of my detention at Port Hedland I was in a bad state emotionally. Most nights I would lie in bed feeling nervous wondering about what would happen to us... Our sleep was also disturbed by the guards checking on us every night. They would open the doors and make sure that everyone was asleep in their rooms.

During the last couple of months of the five and a half years we spent in detention we were really depressed as we heard that the Australian government was going to send us back to Cambodia. Mentally we felt sick and had no lawyers and no one else we could talk to about how we felt. I was so depressed at the time that I had nightmares every night. I also had headaches worrying about what might happen to us and these would last for days. Things would upset me very easily, I could not control my emotions and my anger. I took medicine like sleeping pills and anti-depressants for my problems but this didn't help me. I took medication every night for the last few months I was in detention. I was bored and nervous as I didn't know what would happen. I had no one to talk to. I would spend a lot of my time just looking around and looking up at the sky.

(Human Rights and Equal Opportunity Commission 1999 pp. 229-30)

Family support for children seeking asylum

The family is the basic unit of society and responsible for providing the necessary stable environment to enable the best interests of the child to be maintained. Children do not develop in isolation: effective family functioning is critical in providing the sense of self-esteem, security and identity that is necessary for the child to successfully develop and adapt to the social environment (Almqvist & Broberg 1999). 'The absence of stable family and peer support has been found to be a major predictor of poor psychological adaptation' (Jupp & Luckey 1990).

Refugees' psychosocial well-being is as important as their physical health. The ability of traumatised refugee children to cope with the distressing experiences of war-related and displacement experiences is greatly enhanced by a supportive family and community milieu, one in which parents can continue to project a sense of stability, permanence, and competence to their children. Unless parents are supported to deal with their own trauma and grief they will struggle to provide appropriate support to their children (Ajdukovic 1993; Athey & Ahearn 1991).

While the practice of parenting is culturally bound, some level of routine and parental setting of boundaries broadly characterises normal childhood development. Effective parenting cannot occur in an environment where family and parent-child routines are not possible and where parents' ability to provide a safe and supportive environment critical to children's development is removed. Parents report feeling a lack of control over everyday situations. Life is run by rules and regimentation, even the children's food is prepared by strangers: this erodes family structure where traditional patterns of food preparation, eating and parental role modelling are replaced by the life of the institution (Rogalla & Highfield 2001). Children must queue for food with the adults, be scanned for concealed metal cutlery, and eat what is prepared. The eating times dictated by the detention centre staff often do not fit with the needs of small children. Loss of control of the type of food available and the timing of feeding their children causes distress to mothers, especially when lack of access to food and cooking facilities means they are unable to provide for their children in the ways which they are accustomed to. Small problems can become more significant than if they were within a normal community situation (Pittaway & Bartolomei 2001).

Parents frequently feel shame about the situation their family is in. The feeling of shame among detainees intensifies the severity and instability of family relationships within detention. It is common for men to have strong feelings of shame in front of their own children and wives, not only that they have lost control and power over their current situation but because they often feel responsible for the family's predicament. Their parental roles are affected as they can no longer provide for and protect their families. This seems to be especially strong when detainees them-selves are well educated and once held important occupations. Multiple stressors, such as conflict, violence, marital and familial role breakdown, and severe psychological pressure are likely to produce 'dysfunctional' families. Detention centres appear to be a breeding ground for these stress factors (Pittaway & Maksimovic 2000).

The Human Rights and Equal Opportunity Commission indicates that the boredom and frustration of prolonged detention is apparent in the frequency of violence. They state that the incident reports record a high level of violence and that the counselling required to assist families in coping with their circumstances in detention is not available.

> I am concerned about the length of detention. My husband used to be very kind to us but because of the length of detention he has turned nasty. He is not sleeping till 3.00–4.00am and he is very short tempered with us. He cannot sleep because of the boredom. There is not much room to walk very far from here. I am also worried about the children's education and their future. My husband reckons that we will just die here in detention. We have lost hope.
>
> (Human Rights and Equal Opportunity Commission 1999 p. 233)

> The emotional wellbeing of children is influenced by the protection and care they receive from their families and communities. Adults often suffer greatly in refugee situations; and this can influence their ability to provide for their children. Sometimes parental distress results in child abuse, abandonment, family strife and other forms of family disintegration.
>
> (UNHCR 1994 p. 38)

The experiences of refugee women not only present severe obstacles to their successful resettlement in a country of asylum, they can impact on their ability to respond to the trauma experienced by their children. The often traumatised mothers have to respond to the needs of their children as well as their own requirements to heal and develop coping strategies that will help them support their children. The fact that refugee children and young people are often dependent on adults who are themselves traumatised, and unable to meet the developmental needs of their children, makes them particularly vulnerable to mental health problems (Grunbaum 1997).

A detention centre is not an environment conducive to normal family functioning. There are numerous stressors that affect the family dynamics while in detention, which contribute to the breakdown of family units. It is common for husbands and wives to be separated. There is no current capacity within the detention centres in Australia to separate families from the general population (Rayner 2001) so that families, women, children, young people, and adult males are placed together in common areas. This limits both the privacy and the protection of vulnerable and traumatised women, children and young people, and exacerbates feelings of insecurity and mistrust. Research indicates that children as young as one are able to detect and react to parental distress and that their mental health may be adversely affected (Australian Joint Standing Committee on Social Issues (JSCSI) 1997). Although it is common for parents to shield their children from the reality of their situation, children are often aware of what is going on around them and are anxious about their situation. Children react strongly to being detained and often do not understand why their parents are unable to get the family out of detention. There are reports of children asking their parents what they have done wrong and why they are being 'locked up' and 'punished'. They become frustrated and can not understand why their parents are not protecting them (Pittaway & Maksimovic 2000).

Unaccompanied minors

Unaccompanied children are particularly vulnerable, with the highest mortality in children in refugee camps occurring among the unaccompanied (Murray et al. 2002). They are subject to all the stressors described above but in addition, lack parental and family support. On arrival in Australia they become wards of the Minister for Immigration. There has been some discussion about the potential conflict of interest when responsibility for ensuring the best interests of the child and enforcing a policy of

deterrence towards asylum seekers rests with
ever, there has been no change in this dual
have been held in detention for months, s
released either singly or in small groups a
themselves, with the ad hoc support of
(Uniting Care Burnside 2002).

On arrival they often require assistance tracing
their communities. They need to establish whether their pa...
or dead. They need to let their parents and family know that they are s...
if this can be done without putting their families in danger from authorities because they have aided their escape. Delays in fulfilling these tasks can
compound feelings of fear and anxiety that these young people are already
experiencing. It is part of our obligations under the Refugee Convention
and the Convention of the Rights of the Child that we offer these children an environment of safety and security whether they are allowed to
stay in Australia or not. Detention centres do not provide this opportunity.

Literature reviews and structured interviews with key service providers
indicate that children's experience in detention results in long-term negative impacts when they enter their new community and do not have the
ability to trust people in authority or those who are trying to help them
(Mitchell 2001; Pittaway & Breen 1999). It is reported that even when
clients have learnt to trust health practitioners, advocates or legal advisers,
these service providers are seen as powerless in the face of detention
centre staff and government officials. Withdrawal, suspicion, and loss of
confidence in potential help intensifies the longer people are left in
detention and is often grounded in lived experience. Many workers are
unable to help at anything but a superficial level. People can only regain
the capacity to learn to trust again if they encounter consistent, safe and
benign human relationships, and are presented with some hope for a safe
and secure future (Becker & Silove, cited in Crock 1993 p. 87).

Seeking solutions

The available research and anecdotal evidence from a wide range of
informed and reliable sources clearly demonstrates that prolonged periods
in detention can only serve to exacerbate the trauma of refugees. Advocates in Australia have proposed alternative models to detention. The current evidence, with respect to the negative and compounding impact that
detention has on already traumatised refugees, points to the urgency with
which these alternatives must be considered.

has been argued that there are better, more economically viable and ore humane ways of processing the claims of onshore asylum seekers. In Sweden no child under 18 years is held in detention for more than three days; in extreme circumstances this can be extended to six days (Mitchell 2001). Unaccompanied minors are taken directly to a supervised group home run by the Migration Board and Child Social Services where they undergo medical and psychological assessment and are allocated a caseworker who guides them through the asylum application and settlement procedures. These caseworkers are social workers, counsellors, and people with experience working in closed institutions, bringing sensitivity and experience to their work with asylum seekers (Mitchell 2001).

There have been calls in Australia for the release of all women and children to be allowed to live in the local community under house detention, with visiting rights to family members, in particular fathers who may still be held in detention. This is similar to a Swedish model based on the principle of balancing the sovereign right to border control and protection of one's national interest, with the right of people to seek asylum and the principle of family unity and integrity (Mitchell 2001). In Sweden only those people who may have a criminal record or some other strong reason as to why they should not be released into the community are detained. If males in a family unit are detained, women and children are allowed to live freely in the community; detention centres are in urban areas near to supportive ethnic communities; and during the day, there is open access at the detention centre for families to visit their husbands, fathers, and other family members (Mitchell 2001).

This is not an ideal situation. Research into the long-term recovery of children who survived the Holocaust demonstrates that children who remained with both parents, even in horrendous situations, recovered from the experience better than children who were separated from their parents for what was perceived as their own good (Kinzie 1988). These findings are supported by studies conducted with unaccompanied Vietnamese and Cambodian youth (Felsman et al. 1990; Kinzie 1988; Kinzie et al. 1989). There is a danger that a focus on the needs of children in detention independent of the needs of the family might lead to a situation whereby children are separated from their parents and placed with foster parents or in institutions outside the detention centre. This would be detrimental to the future development of the children and to the capability and functioning of the family units.

A limited trial of removing women and children from the detention centres has begun at Woomera, one of the detention centres in the South Australian desert. The women and children remain under 24 hour surveillance, they can only leave their place of residence under escort of a guard, and visiting times at the detention centre are limited. While it removes them from the situation within the detention camp it splits families that are already traumatised. Another major issue is that Woomera is very isolated and very far from the ethnic communities who could provide much needed emotional support and assistance to the women and children. However, this trial has not yet been evaluated. Indicators for evaluation need to include the policy outcomes such as the ability of the program to provide easy access to the asylum seekers and the comparative cost of community versus institutional detention to be assessed as well as outcomes for the asylum seekers in terms of health and well-being.

It would not be unreasonable to presume that most asylum seekers would have a legitimate claim unless otherwise demonstrated through the screening process. As such it is critical that all measures be taken that may assist in reducing trauma and distress, including the processing of all claims as a matter of urgency and increased service provision to detainees including access to regular medical attention, trauma counselling, early childhood specialists and teachers, appropriate education and activity.

In other Western countries such as Sweden, asylum seekers are given information and services to help them process their applications and begin the slow process of healing and resettlement. The majority are not held in detention centres, but are offered support to live within the community until their application is decided. They are not sent to geographically isolated areas. The role of counsellors and caseworkers includes providing support if a claim for asylum is rejected. Alternatives are discussed with them, and they are escorted on to the next stage of their journey. Research in Europe has shown that resettled refugees who are well supported integrate quickly into the community with no increase in levels of welfare dependency or crime (Mitchell 2001).

Conclusion

The past decade has seen important shifts in opinion reflected in the literature about working with refugee children who have survived torture and trauma. One of the most important of these relates to the resilience of children (Pittaway & Breen 1999). Until quite recently it was believed that children did not fully experience the negative impact of torture and trauma. It is now recognised that children as young as three experience problems in their psychosocial development if they are not given some extra assistance and support. The notion of resilience now relates more to the ability of refugee children and young people to resume their normal development if they are given early assistance and support to build their protective capacities. Early intervention has been recognised as essential to the prevention of later mental health problems (Punamaki 2001). The major concern with current policies is that they are reactive to global events and the perceived need of the community to have a government that is responsive to concerns about security and border sovereignty. The policies do not take into account the potential longer-term implications for the asylum seekers, a large proportion of whom may be found to have valid claims and will resettle in Australia, and the effects on the broader Australian community. Activities by the HREOC, Detention Advisory Committee and the United Nations High Commissioner for Human Rights continue to monitor the situation. Australia's Commissioner for Human Rights stated:

> Australia has international obligations towards children under the Convention on the Rights of the Child...We are required to treat all children the same irrespective of how they come to Australia. Under Federal legislation and international obligations, the Commission has responsibility for monitoring Australia's compliance with the Convention.
>
> (Ozdowski 2001)

An inquiry into the conditions of children in detention in Australia has just been held. The inquiry considered public submissions and visited major detention centres and facilities. The inquiry covered the conditions under which children are detained, their health and education in detention, and the impact of detention on their well-being. This information will add significantly to our knowledge and understanding of the impacts of detention on families and children. It will provide indicators of the steps that need to be taken to begin to address some of the harm caused by this policy to date.

Recommended reading

Almqvist, K., & Broberg, A.G. (1999) Mental health and social adjustment in young refugee children 3 years after their arrival in Sweden, *Journal of the American Academy of Child and Adolescent Psychiatry*, 38(6): 723–30.

Driver, C. and Beltran, R. (1998) Impact of Refugee trauma on children's occupational role as school students, *Australian Occupational Therapy Journal*, 45: 23–38.

Forbes Martin, S. (1991) *Refugee Women*, Zed Books, London and New Jersey.

Goldson, E. (1996) The effect of war on children, *Child Abuse and Neglect* 20(9): 809–19.

HREOC (2002) National Inquiry into Children in Immigration Detention. http://www.humanrights.gov.au/human_rights/children_detention/submissions.

Pittaway, E. & Breen, C. (1999) *Refugee Children Surviving War, Surviving Peace,* AUSINET report.

Pittaway, E. & Maksimovic, N. (2000) Children in Detention, ANCORW and UNSW Centre for Refugee Research Report.

UNHCR (2002) 'The World of Children at a Glance', http://www.unhcr.ch/children/glance.html.

References

Ajdukovic, D.M. (1993) Psychological Well Being of Refugee Children, *Child Abuse and Neglect,* 17: 843–54.

Allodi, F. (1980a) The psychiatric effects in children and families on victims of political persecution and torture, *Danish Medical Bulletin,* 27(5): 229–31.

Allodi, F. (1980b) *The psychiatric effects of political persecution and torture in children and families of victims,* presented at a colloquium on 'The medical and legal aspects of torture', sponsored by Amnesty International Canada, Francophone section, Montreal.

Almqvist, K. & Broberg, A.G. (1999) Mental health and social adjustment in young refugee children 3 years after their arrival in Sweden, *Journal of the American Academy of Child and Adolescent Psychiatry,* 38(6): 723–30.

Andrews, A.B. & Ben-Arieh, A. (1999) Measuring and Monitoring Children's Well-being across the World, *Social Work,* 44(2): 105–14.

Athey, J.L. & Ahearn, F.L. (1991) The mental health of refugee children: An Overview, In Ahearn, F. & Athey, J. (eds) *Refugee Children: theory, research, and services,* Johns Hopkins University Press, Baltimore, pp. 3–19.

Australia Joint Standing Committee on Social Issues (JSCSI) (1997) *Children of Imprisoned Parents. Written report of evidence provided by Louise Abbott of the Australian Red Cross,* NSW Division to the Committee on Thursday, 6/3/97.

Bender, L.E. (2002) Submission to the National Inquiry into Children in Immigration Detention http://www.humanrights.gov.au/human_rights/children_detention/submissions/bender.html.

Commonwealth Ombudsman (2001), Report of an Own Motion Investigation into the Department of Immigration and Multicultural Affairs' Immigration Detention Centres, Office of the Ombudsman, Canberra, pp. 21.

Crock, M. (1993) *Protection or punishment?: the detention of asylum-seekers in Australia,* Federation Press, Sydney.

Felsman, J.K., Leong, F.T., Johnson, M.C. & Felsman, I.C. (1990) Estimates of psychological distress among Vietnamese refugees: Adolescents, unaccompanied minors and young adults, *Social Science and Medicine,* 31(11): 1251–6.

Flood, A. (2001) *Report of Inquiry into Immigration Detention Procedures,* Canberra.

Forbes Martin, S. (1991) *Refugee Women,* Zed Books, London and New Jersey.

Garbarino, J., Kostelny, K. & Dubrow, N. (1991) What Children can tell us about living in danger, *American Psychologist,* 46: 376–83.

Goldson, E. (1996) The effect of war on children, *Child Abuse and Neglect,* 20(9): 809–19.

Grunbaum, L. (1997) Psychotherapy with children in refugee families who have survived torture: containment and understanding of repetitive behaviours and play, *Journal of Child Psychotherapy*, 23(3): 437–52.

Human Rights and Equal Opportunity Commission (1999) 1998–99 Review of immigration detention centres, In vol. 2001 HREOC, Canberra, pp. Available at: http://www.hreoc.gov.au/pdf/human_rights/asylum_seekers/idc_review.pdf.

Huxstep, M. (2002) Submission to the National Inquiry into Children in Immigration Detention http://www.humanrights.gov.au/human_rights/children_detention/submissions/huxstep.html.

Jupp, J. & Luckey, J. (1990) Educational experiences in Australia of Indo-Chinese adolescent refugees, *International Journal of Mental Health*, 18(4): 78–91.

Kinzie, J.D. (1988) The psychiatric effects of massive trauma on Cambodian refugees, In Wilson, J.P. & Harel, Z. (eds), *Human adaptation to extreme stress: From the Holocaust to Vietnam*, Plenum Press, New York, pp. 305–17.

Kinzie, J.D., Sack, W., Angell, R. & Clarke, G. (1989) A three-year follow-up of Cambodian young people traumatized as children, *Journal of the American Academy of Child and Adolescent Psychiatry*, 28(4): 501–4.

Mitchell, G. (2001) Asylum Seekers in Sweden, An integrated approach to reception, detention, determination, integration and return, In http://www.refugeecouncil.org.au/alternativeSwed.htm.

Molony, J. (2000) Looking at Australia Through Razor Wire, In *Canberra Times*, Canberra.

Murray, C., King, G., Lopez, A., Tomijima, N. & Krug, E. (2002) Armed conflict as a public health problem, *British Medical Journal*, 324: 346–9.

Ozdowski, S. (2001) *National Enquiry into Children in Immigration Detention, November 20* http://www.hreoc.gov.au/media-releases/2001/01_71.html, accessed August 2002.

Peterson, C.C. (1996) *Looking forward through the lifespan: developmental psychology*, Prentice Hall, New York, Sydney.

Pittaway, E. (ed) (1998) Unsung Heroes, *Transcultural Mental Health Journal*, Transcultural Mental Health, Sydney.

Pittaway, E. & Bartolomei, L. (2001) *Fieldwork Notes*, ANCORW and UNSW Centre for Refugee Research Report.

Pittaway, E. & Breen, C. (1999) *Refugee Children, Surviving War, Surviving Peace*, AUSINET Report.

Pittaway, E. & Maksimovic, N. (2000) *Children in Detention*, ANCORW and UNSW Centre for Refugee Research Report.

Punamaki, R.L. (2001) From childhood trauma to adult well-being through psychosocial assistance of Chilean families, *Journal of Community Psychology*, 29(3): 281–303.

Rayner, M. (2001) Political Pinballs: The plight of child refugees in Australia, *Walter Murdoch Lecture*, 31 October 2001, Murdoch University, Perth.

Refugee Council of Australia (2002) The Detention of Asylum Seekers in Europe, available at: http://www.refugeecouncil.org.au/alternativeEurope.htm.

Rogalla, B. & Highfield, T. (2001) The Systematic Incarceration of Children in Immigration Detention Centers of Australia: A Modern Form of Torture, In *OMCT Conference Children, Torture and other Forms of Violence*, Tampere, Finland.

Silove, D., Steel, Z.M. & Watters, C.P. (2000) Policies of Deterrence and the Mental Health of Asylum Seekers, *Journal of the American Medical Association*, 284(5): 604–11.

Sultan, A. & O'Sullivan, K. (2001) Psychological disturbances in asylum seekers held in long term detention: a participant–observer account, *Medical Journal of Australia*, 175: 593–6.

UNHCR (1992) *Guidelines for Educational Assistance to Refugees*, UNHCR, Geneva.

UNHCR (1994) *Refugee Children: Guidelines on Protection and Care*, UNHCR, Geneva.

UNHCR (1995) *Guidelines on Preventing and Responding to Sexual Violence against Refugee Women*, UNHCR, Geneva.

UNHCR (2002) Population Data Unit, March 2002, www.unchr.ch

United Nations (1989) *The Convention on the Rights of the Child*.

United Nations Department of Public Information (1948), Universal Declaration of Human Rights, vol. 2001, United Nations, Geneva.

Uniting Care Burnside (2002) Submission to the National Inquiry into Children in Immigration Detention http://www.humanrights.gov.au/human_rights/children_detention/submissions/bender.html.

Vinson, T. & Lester, E. (1998) A high price for freedom, In *Sydney Morning Herald*, Sydney, p. 22.

West, D. (2000) interview with Dale West Centacare, SA., In *The World Today*, ABC Radio, Adelaide, Dale West interview, 15 November 2000.

7

Refugee Women and Settlement: Gender and Mental Health

Ida Kaplan and Kim Webster

Introduction

The majority of the world's refugees are women and their dependants. UNICEF estimates that over 80 per cent of the refugees resulting from warfare alone are women and children (Brautigam 1996). Ethnic cleansing, massacres, state-sanctioned violence and torture are all weapons in the struggle for power. They are deliberate strategies used to break down communities and their power to resist.

Refugee women facing the tasks of resettlement and adaptation to a new culture may also be survivors of systematic abuse of human rights and dislocation, the consequences of which are widespread, long-term, and potentially trans-generational. Responding to the mental health consequences of experiences of violence and loss, while promoting well-being in the course of settlement, requires addressing fundamental goals. Responses include the provision of safety, the restoration of hope, the building of connections and community strength, and the promotion of human dignity and value. Responding to the multiplicity of mental health needs in a way that meets these conditions requires a practice orientation, which is culturally responsive, gives due consideration to both manifest and less visible difficulties, promotes access, equity and participation, and is committed to increasing the power which women have over their lives in psychological, social and economic terms.

The focus of this chapter is on the impact of pre-arrival experiences and the demands of the settlement process on the mental health of refugee women and their families. Goals to enhance well-being and mental health and how they can be achieved are also presented.

The pre-settlement experience

Over the past fifty years, half a million refugees and displaced persons have resettled in Australia; 48 per cent have been female. The countries of origin of these entrants have changed over the years, reflecting changes in world zones of conflict. In the last ten years, most refugee women have come from Vietnam, Central American countries, the former Yugoslavia, the Horn of Africa region, and Iraq. If the nature of persecution and degree of dislocation were closely examined, differences would emerge in the specific experiences faced by women from different countries. However, horrific violence, extensive loss, being witness to violations on a mass scale and being forced to make impossible choices would be common to most.

The resilience, skills and tenacity needed to survive horrific events and reach Australia after a settlement selection process which excludes so many, testifies to the remarkable adaptiveness of refugees (Silove & Kinzie 2001). The strength of women in this regard requires ongoing acknowledgment. But it is also important to highlight the adverse effects of the refugee experience, because they need to be accommodated when planning appropriate service responses.

Horrific violence, threats to the existence of children, and human rights violations on a mass scale are traumatic events because they can overwhelm the coping capacity of any human being. The Victorian Foundation for Survivors of Torture (VFST) has developed a conceptual framework that links traumatic events to their mental health effects, termed 'the trauma reaction'. The framework is applicable to both genders, but gender-specific causes are highlighted.

The first column in figure 7.1 summarises the acts of persecution and conditions of hardship that characterise refugee experiences before arrival in a settlement country. The second column shows the resulting social and psychological experiences. These are internalised by women, families and communities, and lead to profound effects, some of which can be disabling. These effects on mental health are shown in the third column.

Violent events that refugee women have experienced are rarely isolated incidents. In a climate of political oppression and legitimised brutality, persecution is a daily event, culminating in arrest, sexual slavery, torture, and often death of loved ones. Forced flight from persecution, which results in displacement, severe economic hardship, and lack of access to basic services, continues the perilous circumstances of men, women, and children. Women and their dependants are often separated from the male members of the family, during conflict and in the post-conflict situation leaving

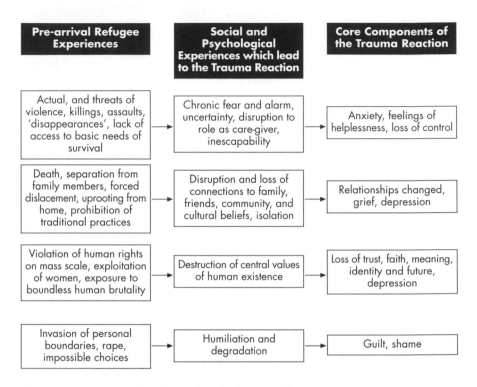

Figure 7.1 Summary of conditions that characterise refugee experiences

them as solely responsible for the security and sustenance of the family. New responsibilities, however, are not matched by the status and rights afforded men, and in many situations women are disadvantaged and made vulnerable as a result. For example, in some refugee camps, food rations are distributed through men. Women may be forced to provide sexual favours to get 'protection' from men and to get food and other essential items in a camp situation.

Women are also subject to the hardships, threats, and violence directed at their children, who are especially vulnerable to prolonged squalor, malnutrition, and continuing exposure to violence in both conflict and post-conflict situations. The mental health effects that result from such experiences, the trauma reaction, can be thought of in terms of symptoms and psychiatric diagnoses and there is certainly evidence of depression and anxiety resulting from war and extreme oppression (Dennersten et al. 1993). Such effects can be measured, but in existential terms, the psychological toll is enormous when there is destruction of the very fabric of life. There are, for example, a host of anxiety symptoms that comprise the psychological sequelae of violence but it is helplessness and loss of control in the face of threat and violence which renders individuals internally powerless and in a chronic state of alarm even once the violence has abated. It is the aim of the oppressor or persecutory regime to break down opposition by creating a state of terror that permeates the family and community as a whole. Women and children are increasingly the targets of persecution because destroying the family structure weakens the entire community, potentially for generations.

Loss characterises the lives of all refugee women; loss of loved ones, loss of home, loss of homeland, loss of identity and perhaps most destructive of all, the loss of the capacity to protect their children and their families. These losses shatter a sense of continuity and identity. Killing, dislocation, and prohibition of traditional practices are some of the ways to achieve this. Other methods are less visible such as creating a climate of suspicion and mistrust to break down social cohesion. Deprivation of basic human rights such as the right to work, education and health, further disrupt a sense of belonging and connectedness. As a result, women, and the community of which they are part, can become passive, depressed, and withdrawn. The destruction of parent-child bonds, is one of the most powerful ways to perpetuate damage, again, across generations.

The witnessing of human rights violations on a mass scale shatters the very assumptions of human existence—the very right to exist can be destroyed because one has been treated as if one is nothing. The meaning of life, god and faith in humanity are all questioned. Women and men of whatever age who have experienced torture and witnessed death and destruction have been exposed to the darkest side of human nature. As Simpson (1993) poignantly wrote of the torture victim, she or he 'confronts the world's loneliness, mercilessness, and nothingness' (p. 153). Shattering previous assumptions of the self and the world lead the victim to more readily accept a submissive position in relation to an oppressor. Justice is no longer expected and yet to counter this destruction, survivors and their communities desperately seek justice and restoration of meaning, a quest which is a strong feature of their adaptation to the post-conflict and settlement environments.

Another legacy of the refugee experience that is critical to recognise is shame and guilt. Humiliation and degradation always accompany acts of violence. Physical boundaries are invaded, the right to privacy is deliberately violated, and the basic functions of eating, sleeping, and going to the toilet are closely controlled. Women particularly are the victims of such violations. They are cursed, degraded, and sexually violated in order to eternally taint them as worthless and discardable. Rape has become a weapon of war and recently recognised as such (United Nations 1993).

Tragically, the power of rape to condemn women to ostracism and isolation and break down the family makes it an effective weapon. 'Rape and sexual abuse is the most common form of systematised torture used against women, and this ranges from gang rape by groups of soldiers, to rape by trained dogs and the brutal mutilation of women's genitalia' (Pittaway et al. 1999). Some refugees who have arrived in Australia have reported that in the concentration camps of Bosnia, family members were forced to perpetrate rape on one another and commit other unspeakable atrocities. Such acts are designed to permanently taint survivors with shame and guilt.

Guilt is also induced by confronting women with impossible choices. It is an excruciating reality for many women that they have had to leave children behind in the hope of future reunion. Other women have to take up a resettlement offer while a spouse is still missing. Even though it may have been impossible to act differently, many women retain the belief that they should have done more to help others. Guilt can be so great that their identity as mothers is destroyed. Certainly, both guilt and shame can weaken the capacity of women to fight back long after they arrive in Australia.

Settlement and mental health

The quality of the settlement environment has the power to mitigate the traumatic effects of violence and human rights violations or the demands of settlement can also exacerbate the legacy of violence just described. Refugee women face multiple adjustment tasks associated with settlement and long-term effects on mental health ultimately depend on an interaction between pre-arrival experiences and the way settlement demands are met. Figure 7.2 shows the link between settlement experiences and components of the trauma reaction.

Serious threats to women can persist in the new settlement environment, particularly when family members remain exposed to danger in the country of origin. Countries from which women come often continue to be war zones. Anxiety about the welfare of family members and friends left behind therefore continues and maintains a sense of powerlessness and anxiety. Guilt is also intensified as a result of having left family members behind. An unfamiliar environment and the disruptive effects of symptoms create further anxiety about ever regaining control and engender great uncertainty about the future. Racist based attacks are another significant source of anxiety. Attacks against Muslim women in the Australian community escalated following the terrorist attacks in the US on 11 September 2001. They became targets because they are a visible minority.

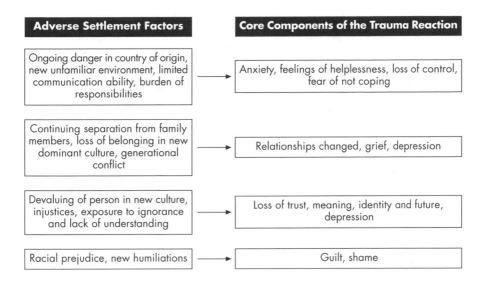

Figure 7.2 Link between settlement experience and trauma reaction

Such attacks have seriously eroded the safety of their everyday environment and constitute serious humiliations.

Dislocation from their own culture and confrontation with a different dominant culture is a challenging process for refugee women. Adjustment to an entirely different system of law, education, and health services is not easily made and conflict and tension can result from a clash in cultural values. There are different responses to the demands of acculturation. Some women move towards incorporating new values whereas others have no hesitation in rejecting the unfamiliar.

Daily activities can present major stressors for refugee women including engagement with the education system with their children. It is women who enrol their children in schools, which is an unfamiliar environment for some families who may never have had the opportunity to provide education for their children. Some common fears that parents have expressed in school based support groups conducted for parents and primary school aged children are: the fear that children may be taken away, the fear that children will not follow their parents' values, the fear that traditions will be lost and the fear that the perceived *laissez-faire* discipline in schools will fail to educate their children (Victorian Foundation for Survivors of Torture (VFST) 2002). These fears are understandable considering previous lack of capacity to provide essential needs for their children.

Isolation, which compounds fear, is a major problem for women. Other refugees from the same community can provide critically important support given the ongoing level of loss and disconnection but they can also remind the person of earlier trauma or represent an ongoing threat if they are perceived as being linked to perpetrators (Daniel & Knudsen 1995).

The sense of isolation can extend to the family domain. Women have to sustain their role of caring for others—their partners, members of the extended family and children—without their own parents who rarely accompany them to Australia (Athey & Ahearn 1991). Isolation also comes from the breakdown in family relationships. Mothers become disempowered by the fact that children often carry the role of communication with institutions and service providers. They also face the fact that their children adapt more quickly than themselves (Klimidis & Minas 1995). Generational conflict arises between mothers and adolescents who want to embrace different values (Nguyen & Williams 1989).

The most destructive impact on women and the family, is domestic violence. Peavey and Zarkovic (1996), writing about women refugees in Bosnia, poignantly described the impact of war on family violence.

> For the women on all sides, the war has marched through their own living rooms. The men in their lives…have brought their brutality and addictions home. Family violence has risen markedly. On all sides of the war, men, if they are lucky enough to come home, have returned bearing guns and internal wounds which are now directed at the women who must live with them (p. 15).

The extent to which men's experiences of being victims of violence contribute to violence against women, compared with long-standing inequities regarding power and privilege, and accepted cultural or religious traditions, is difficult to ascertain. It is known that violence against women cuts across lines of income, class, and culture (Australian Office for the Status of Women 2001; Brautigam 1996) and there is no data to show that the prevalence of family violence is greater among refugee women than women who are not refugees. Without knowing the relative weight of the various causal factors for gender-based violence, it is nevertheless reasonable to assert that the risk factors would be high for refugee women.

In the home, the effects of family violence, which extends to economic deprivation, are extensive. The consequences for the woman include anxiety, depression, humiliation, apathy, psychosomatic symptoms, lowered self-esteem, alcoholism, and suicide (Gulcur 2000). For the family, safety, trust, and affiliative connections are eroded.

The role changes within the family, which accompany the settlement process, can also constitute significant stress for women. Women arriving as sole parents are forced to face new roles and responsibilities such as single parent child rearing. In some situations they become the breadwinner even if they have arrived with a partner. The loss of face and self-esteem for the husband can lead to considerable tension and conflict because of their feelings of helplessness.

Women have the major responsibility for establishing the home and carrying out domestic duties. As for women from non-refugee backgrounds, aspirations for education, training, employment, and social activities create extra demands and pressures when child care and household duties are not shared. Role overload and conflict are associated with psychological distress (McBride 1989; Ross & Mirowsky 1983). In some situations role changes within the family are beneficial. Many women enjoy their newly found rights and have changed the power relationship in families for the better. Further, where household responsibilities are shared, training and education opportunities can lead to higher self-esteem.

There are other settlement needs that influence the well-being of women. They are the importance of finding suitable accommodation and communication. However, the process of satisfying these basic needs is often fraught with problems.

> Nadereh had been detained and tortured. Part of her torture was to watch women being immersed in acid. She herself had had boiling water poured on her. She arrived in Australia with two children, her husband had been executed. Amongst the multiple needs was housing. She would reject house after house, much to the chagrin of housing workers. The reason was that she sought a house full of light. All the houses had reminded her of her detention and torture. Eventually, such a house was found with considerable advocacy which alerted housing service providers to Nadereh's special needs.
>
> (VFST case example)

The search for suitable housing is complicated by a number of factors, other than issues of torture and trauma. Affordable housing is in short supply, accommodation for large families is especially limited and some families face discrimination by real estate agents (Campbell 1997).

The ability to communicate is fundamental to the settlement process. However, there are particular barriers for women in language acquisition: many women cannot get to English classes because of the need to care for young children; the classes are mixed and the presence of men in the classroom prohibits some women from attending for cultural and religious reasons; some women may be afraid of men because of violence perpetrated against them by men and others are not accustomed to expressing their opinions in public.

In highlighting the common issues that affect the mental health of refugee women, one still needs to maintain responsiveness to diversity as a result of differences in degree of exposure to traumatic events, education, religion, and history. A woman from a village who is illiterate, has never been to a city, and whose country has been under siege for twenty years has different needs from a woman who is educated, familiar with urban life, and recently dislocated. Nevertheless for all women there are multiple layers of what could be considered risk factors to mental health. Social networks, personal resources, and family support that would generally be protective are usually limited. Many of the issues raised also apply to other population groups who are disadvantaged; survivors of chronic abuse, or who have a minority status in society.

Principles and strategies for addressing mental health issues

Promoting psychosocial health for women requires balancing a public mental health approach, with its emphasis on health promotion and early intervention, with a focus on women with existing poor mental health who require intensive attention. Further, the multiple determinants of health provide a very wide range of possibilities for intervention (Victorian Health Promotion Foundation 2000).

Interventions can be conceptualised as addressing needs that have been frequently identified (Clinton-Davis & Fassil 1992; National Forum of Services for Survivors of Torture and Trauma (NFSSTT) 1999; Pittaway 1991) and highlighted above. An alternative conceptualisation is to group or analyse needs in a way that reflects the legacy of the refugee experience. As outlined in the above sections, refugee women have had their power and control eroded for many years, their relationships with family and community have been threatened and destroyed to varying degrees and their dignity and value as human beings has been undermined. Accordingly, needs are for empowerment and control, restoration of relationships and restoration of meaning, dignity and value. Figure 7.3 summarises strategies that could enhance women's mental health.

Enhancing and restoring control

A secure environment with adequate provision and access to health, welfare, education, and accommodation are among the most basic needs of refugee women. All women refugees have been subject to deprivation in these areas and it is the responsibility of service providers and workers to facilitate access to relevant services and maximise choice. Each service area deserves extended discussion regarding ways to maximise choice and

Enhancing control
- promoting access
- information provision
- integrated service provision, i.e. integration of mental health services into general health services
- 'exploiting' the reciprocal relationship among women's health, children's health, and men's health

Restoring connections
- group participation: recreational, story-writing, information sharing and provision
- linking with supportive groups and agencies
- information dissemination and participation through media
- community education covering topics of interest: role of women in Australian society, communication patterns in dominant culture
- participation in training and educational programs and employment
- strengthening families
- community building
- a trusting, continuing connection with an available caring adult
- intensive support, i.e. counselling/advocacy

Restoring dignity and value
- upholding human rights
- reducing racism and discrimination
- participation in decision making
- quality of care

Figure 7.3 Strategies for promoting and improving mental health in refugee women

control. As a comprehensive coverage is not possible within the scope of this chapter, the issue of access is highlighted because it is central to the experience of safety, predictability, and control.

Access to services requires active promotion and overcoming of barriers, the most important of which is the language barrier. A number of interpreting services operate in the states and territories; however the need exceeds available resources. Even where resources are adequate, service providers may underutilise interpreters because they are not familiar themselves with methods of access and booking interpreters.

Facilitating communication and language acquisition can be enhanced by:
- adequate interpreting resources
- offering flexible language training options such as women–only classes and home-based tuition
- providing language training as part of established women's social/ recreational groups
- arrangements for more flexible tuition and a generous 'window period' for women with difficulty learning due to trauma effects and for women who are illiterate
- overcoming practical barriers such as child-care and geographical location

The importance of language acquisition is recognised by the Australian Government through funding for the Adult Migration Education Program (AMEP) to deliver 510 hours of English tuition for newly arrived humanitarian entrants. In 1997 additional funding became available for the delivery of special preparatory programs of up to 100 hours for the special learning needs of refugees.

Information provision about services and professionals who are culturally responsive is one of the strategies to enhance access. In itself, information is an empowering tool because it increases choice and familiarity with new systems. For example, knowing who is a 'bulk-billing' general practitioner, who speaks their language or uses interpreters, has obvious value. Torture and trauma services, in collaboration with community health centres in some instances, orient new arrivals to the Australian health care system and the range of health-related services (National Forum of Services for Survivors of Torture and Trauma (NFSSTT) 1999). It is vital to anticipate the familiarity and acceptability of the information being offered. It is relatively straightforward to describe services and how to reach them, but information about child protection issues or health issues such as female genital mutilation require information provision to be part of broader community education strategies.

Despite the obvious importance of information provision, there are a number of issues to be considered when planning and implementing its delivery:

- the best setting for information provision re access
- comparing the benefits of face-to-face delivery with provision of translated materials
- the relevance of providing information that is tailored to individual circumstances.
- the amount and rate at which information is presented so that it can be absorbed
- the likely familiarity or novelty of the information
- inclusion of information about their rights as service users
- establishing the credentials of the organisation providing the information, i.e. relationship to other government departments, experience with refugees, political affiliations/neutrality

Finally, access to services would best be achieved through integration of services. The reciprocal relationship among women's health, children's health and men's health can be 'exploited'. The first point of contact for a refugee family using mainstream services may be a man seeking physical health care from a general practitioner. This can lead the general practitioner to explore the health of all family members. Once appointments are made with other family members, links to other appropriate services can be made. Similarly, information about children's educational needs, provided in a school setting, can lead to information about availability of and nature of health services in the local area.

Integration of mental health care into general health care is another way to enhance access and has numerous advantages. Stigma associated with mental health problems can be avoided. Further, in the health context, psychological problems that are experienced, or presented as somatic symptoms can be attended to. Follow-up of women and their families is also ensured. A holistic approach to mental health that recognises that psychological health depends in part on physical health means that attention to the special health issues of women will also benefit their mental health. Family planning, quality care for pregnancies, and treatment of gynaecological problems and sexually transmitted diseases are also opportunities to benefit the psychological well-being of women. For many refugee women health care in these areas is especially salient because their health problems are intimately connected with traumatic events. For example, pregnancy and sexually transmitted diseases may have resulted from rape.

Restoring connections

Multiple sources of support can be fostered among friends, the host community, and the woman's community. Enabling refugee women to support one another is critical so that they are active agents of change, not passive recipients of help (Dankelman et al. 1988). Several initiatives have brought women together and established ongoing networks such as the Victorian Network on Refugee Women's Issues (Couch 1997).

Gender role expectations affect opportunities for participation. Some of the factors previously described as influencing English class attendance apply to other contexts as well. Women from some backgrounds cannot participate in a mixed gender environment, or their participation is hindered by their fears of men. These factors would have implications for organising orientation programs, support groups, and recreation programs. Several programs have been developed which enable women to attend women-only groups.

Where social contact and participation is the central aim of programs, trauma effects need to be considered. To allow for fear of renewed loss, distrust, feelings of anger and shame, social contact should be structured so that there is room for withdrawal as well as opportunities for the gradual development of trust.

Ethnic community support services and programs that link women to their communities have the advantage of enabling the development of relationships with undue barriers due to distrust. The voluntary sector has provided great support to women in the way of reducing isolation and offering practical family support (Nsubage-Kyobe & Dimock 2000).

A number of programs have been developed in Australia to assist the settlement of refugee women and their families. Consultations with women have contributed to the content of programs, which in many cases are led or co-facilitated by refugee women. The programs include: Families in Cultural Transition produced by the Service for the Treatment and Rehabilitation of Torture and Trauma Survivors (STARTTS New South Wales 1996), which has been adapted for use by various organisations including the Voiceless Children's Network in conjunction with the Inner West Migrant Resource Centre, New South Wales.

Contributing to the well-being of all members of the family unit is critical to women's recovery from trauma associated with the refugee experience. Strengthening families by providing support to all members and ensuring that family members are assisted in facing major transitions to new environments are of course important goals in themselves.

Given the findings that parental responsiveness, emotional stability of families and the mental health of mothers affects the mental health of children (Raundelen 1993), supporting women in their role as mothers will positively influence the mental health of children. Effective support can be indirect, using the various strategies that address a range of settlement needs. But specific strategies are also needed to assist mothers to deal with their emotional problems and the impact of traumatic experiences on their children. Relevant skills include modelling constructive coping behaviour (Dankelman et al. 1988; Garbarino & Kostelny 1993; Garbarino et al. 1991a, b), ways to respond to increased arousal, reactivity to reminders of past events and behavioural regression in children; and legitimising the child's emotional responses. Mothers of young infants particularly require emotional support, because of their vulnerability to extreme isolation and depression (Pittaway 1991).

A number of parenting programs have been developed that provide specific guidelines on how to deal with traumatic reactions and other stress reactions in children (Drygevrov & Raundelen 1998; Raundelen 1993). Assistance has to be offered sensitively because recognition of a child's problems is difficult for a mother, possibly shattering expectations that life in a new country will put an end to terrible events of the past and their impact on children. Sensitive assistance also means that any guidance should occur in the context of an established relationship with a trusted person or group of people and preferably be part of an intervention program with additional, broader aims. This would allow mothers to approach the issue of child trauma with some control over how much they are ready to 'take in'. The level of assistance given is therefore guided by need as perceived by the woman.

Where trauma has been prolonged and women suffer persistent disabling symptoms or they and their families are at risk of deterioration in their level of functioning, intensive support in the form of individually tailored advocacy and counselling is required. Such support is provided by torture and trauma services and other agencies such as community health centres and sexual assault clinics.

Assessment underpins choosing the best way to assist. A holistic approach to assessment is required. This means that a range of needs are screened for and some formulation is made regarding causes of difficulties that can be psychological, biological, social, and practical. It is important through the process of assessment to enquire about needs, beyond the presenting ones, as they will not necessarily be raised.

To be comprehensive, this usually takes time and where the encounter is a brief one, the presenting difficulty may have to be taken at face value. Nevertheless, good background knowledge of a country, familiarity with its cultural and religious diversity, and familiarity with the history of conflict and oppression in the region does enable reasonable assumptions to be made about a woman's needs. Where needs are complex, it is expected that a woman may be dependent on an agency for assistance. However, it is important to foster independence in the long run by assisting with developing a social support network, building skills and confidence, and by reducing the intensity of symptoms that interfere with everyday functioning.

> A client of the VFST was a young mother who was very anxious and grieving for the loss of her son who was killed during the war in Bosnia. She was 8 months pregnant and extremely worried about the imminent birth of her baby, because she feared another loss. Having recently arrived in Australia it was critical to introduce her to the medical system in Australia so that she would know what to expect as well as inform the hospital of her situation. Assistance was also provided in regard to finding suitable accommodation. Relatively soon after the birth of her baby she felt able to make appointments herself, felt comfortable doing so and was actively seeking suitable housing. Subsequently she was able to talk about her grief over her first son's death.
>
> (VFST case example)

Advocacy and counselling were part of the intensive support provided. For some clients, the concept of counselling is an unfamiliar and unacceptable one and there is often a preference not to disclose material that is distressing. Alternative means of assistance, are extremely important in such cases. These can include: natural therapies, linking the woman to agencies that provide emotional support as part of their service to clients, intensive practical support such as accompanying clients to appointments, which also allows for discussion of general concerns, and linking the woman to traditional healers.

A problem that requires intensive support is that of family violence. Studies in a number of countries of resettlement suggest that the legal prohibition of domestic violence and an active law enforcement approach has a powerful deterrent effect. Nevertheless what is enshrined in law can be difficult to uphold when it clashes with different values about acceptable disciplinary methods and openness to public scrutiny of family matters. Other factors that limit choices for refugee women who are victims of domestic violence, are lack of an extended family network for support, wariness of police and judicial authorities who may be associated with state sanctioned violence in their countries of origin, cultural prohibitions against separation and divorce, and pressure to keep the family together, given trauma and dislocation suffered.

Restoring dignity and value

All the strategies described thus far contribute to restoring dignity and value. When consciousness about the importance of dignity informs the development of ways to contribute to the well-being of refugee women, methods of implementation are likely to be appropriate and respectful of women's rights.

Foremost to restoring dignity is the recognition that refugee women offer unique and valuable qualities to receiving societies and bring important resources to the task of settlement. The experience of international aid organisations is that refugee women are key contributors to community and economic development initiatives in refugee and other emergency situations. This involvement testifies not only to the skills and attributes of refugee women, but also to their survival skills and motivation in conditions of adversity. In countries of settlement refugee women have demonstrated a preparedness to organise both with one another and with women in their wider community to share common experiences and address problems of violence and gender inequality. This has contributed to mutual understanding and harmony among refugee communities and between those communities and the wider society.

Alongside recognition of women's resources, ensuring the dignity of all women still requires changes at the broadest level. Many refugee women come from countries where gender inequality was the norm. Refugee women may be less likely than their male counterparts to be literate, to be educated, or to have an established work history, all of which put them at some disadvantage for accessing settlement resources, specialist services, and participating in language and orientation programs. Strategies for building gender equity and reducing discrimination against women are therefore crucial.

Restoring dignity also means wide public recognition of human rights violations and deprivations experienced, restitution, and social justice. In post-conflict situations, tribunals and commissions such as the International Criminal Tribunal for the Former Yugoslavia and the Truth and Reconciliation Commission in South Africa provide a platform for the telling of people's stories so that there is a witnessing process for victims. In countries of resettlement a process for affirmation of the suffering of the victim is also needed. This has taken place through dissemination of women's stories and special community events that highlight the experiences of women. Much more could be done in this regard to ensure that women receive public recognition of their experiences and that their experiences are understood. Every survivor struggles to find meaning in their suffering and many women have done so by bearing witness to their experiences. This endeavour should be supported and encouraged where possible through participation in socio-political action, and projects which have as their aim expression of the struggle.

Finally, there is an opportunity to build dignity with every human encounter. Given that it is the human hand that has perpetrated violations it is the human hand that has the power to heal wounds. The quality of relationships can however, be undermined when workers face the sheer immensity of needs. To deal with being potentially overwhelmed, overly distant styles of working can occur, whereby women's problems are minimised or overlooked. Alternatively, some workers respond with 'rescuing' that diminishes the power of women. Awareness of such responses and the implications for ways of working require sufficient levels of support and professional development.

Conclusion

The well-being and mental health of refugee women and their families requires the facilitation of their settlement while recognising the legacy of their experiences prior to their arrival in Australia. Strategies are needed that support their access to social and economic resources such as employment, education and recreation, their equal participation in civic life and their freedom from violence in both the public and private realms. Intensive support is required for those women and family members suffering severe adverse psychological effects from traumatic events.

Failure to act in these areas isolates women survivors of torture and trauma and robs them of a future. Without adequate support for the settlement process they are vulnerable to psychological disorders and it means that they will have suffered for nothing.

Public policy recognises gender inequities and upholds rights to access and culturally responsive service provision. A holistic framework for understanding needs and planning ways to address those needs is increasingly the norm. However, needs far outstrip resources and it is a challenge to maintain a balance between mental health promotion, prevention, and intervention.

Recommended reading

Bemak, F., Chung R.C.-Y. & Pedersen, P. (2002) *Counselling refugees: a psychosocial approach to innovative multicultural interventions*, Greenwood Publishing Press.

UNHCR & Victorian Foundation for Survivors of Torture (VFST) (2002) *Refugee resettlement: an international handbook to guide reception and integration*, UNHCR, Geneva.

Victorian Foundation for Survivors of Torture (1998) *Rebuilding Shattered Lives*. (Guide to those working with the survivors of torture and trauma.), VFST, Melbourne.

References

Athey, J.L. & Ahearn, F.L. (1991) The mental health of refugee children: An Overview, In Ahearn, F. & Athey, J. (eds), *Refugee Children: theory, research, and services*, Johns Hopkins University Press, Baltimore, pp. 3–19.

Australian Office for the Status of Women (2001) *Working Together Against Violence: The first three years of partnerships against domestic violence*, Commonwealth of Australia.

Brautigam, C.A. (1996) Traumatized Women: Overcoming victimization through equality and non-discrimination, In Danieli, Y., Rodley, N.S. & Weisath, L. (eds), *International Responses to Traumatic Stress*, Baywood, New York, pp. 347–66.

Campbell, S.D. (1997) Housing Needs of Refugees, *National Network of Refugee Women's Issues Newsletter*, 9: 14–15.

Clinton-Davis, L. & Fassil, Y. (1992) Health and Social Problems of Refugees, *Social Science & Medicine*, 35: 507–13.

Couch, J. (1997) New Network of Refugee Women, *National Network of Refugee Women's Issues Newsletter*, 9: 18.

Daniel, V. & Knudsen, J.C. (eds) (1995) *Mistrusting Refugees*, University of California Press, Berkeley.

Dankelman, I., Davidson, J. & International Union for Conservation of Nature and Natural Resources (1988) *Women and environment in the Third World: alliance for the future*, Earthscan Pub., in association with IUCN.

Dennersten, L., Astbury, J. & Morse, C. (1993) *Psychosocial and Mental Health Aspects of Women's Health*, World Health Organisation, Geneva.

Drygevrov, A. & Raundelen, M. (1998) *Advising Parents of Refugee Children*, Centre for Crisis Psychology, Bergen.

Garbarino, J. & Kostelny, K. (1993) Children's response to war: What do we know?, In Leavitt, L.A. & Fox (eds), *Psychological Effects of War and Violence on Children*, Lawrence Erlbaum, Hillsdale.

Garbarino, J., Kostelny, K. & Dubrow, N. (1991a) *No Place to be a child: Growing up in a War Zone*, Lexington.

Garbarino, J., Kostelny, K. & Dubrow, N. (1991b) What Children can tell us about living in danger, *American Psychologist*, 46: 376–83.

Gulcur, L. (2000) Evaluating the Role of Gender Inequalities and Rights Violations. *Women's Mental Health, Health and Human Rights: An International Journal*, 5: 46–67.

Klimidis, S. & Minas, I.H. (1995) Migration, culture and mental health in children and adolescents, In Guerra, C. & White, R. (eds), *Ethnic Minority Youth*, National Clearinghouse for Youth Studies, Hobart.

McBride, A.B. (1989) Multiple Roles and Depression, *Health Values*, 13: 45–9.

National Forum of Services for Survivors of Torture and Trauma (NFSSTT) (1999) *A Sound Investment: A report of the progress of the National Early Intervention program for refugee and humanitarian program entrants*, NFSSTT, Canberra.

Nguyen, N.A. & Williams, H.L. (1989) Transition from East to West: Vietnemese Adolescents and Their Parents, *Journal of American Academy of Child and Adolescent Psychiatry*, 28: 505–15.

Nsubage-Kyobe, A. & Dimock, L. (2000) *African Communities and Settlement Services in Victoria: Towards Best Practice Service Delivery Models*, Department of Immigration and Multicultural and Indigenous Affairs, Australia.

Peavey, F. & Zarkovic, R.M. (1996) *I remember: Writings by Bosnian Women Refugees*, Lute Books, San Francisco.

Pittaway, E. (1991) *Refugee women still at risk in Australia: a study of the first two years of resettlement in the Sydney Metropolitan Area*, AGPS, Canberra.

Pittaway, E., Ferguson, B. & Transcultural Mental Health Centre (1999) Refugee Women—The Unsung Heroes, Nobody wants to talk about it: refugee women's mental health, *Current issues in transcultural mental health*, Conference Publications, Springwood, NSW, pp. ix, 114.

Raundelen, M. (1993) *Family and War: Some observations and suggestions for further research*, paper presented at the Third European Conference on Traumatic Stress, Bergen.

Ross, C.E. & Mirowsky, J. (1983) Child Care and Adjustment to Wives' Employment, *Journal of Health and Social Behaviour*, 29: 127–38.

Service for the Treatment and Rehabilitation of Torture and Trauma Survivors (STARTTS NSW) (1996), *Families in Cultural Transition—A resource kit, New Connections*, STARTTS NSW, Sydney.

Silove, D. & Kinzie, J.D. (2001) Survivors of war trauma, mass violence, and civilian terror, In Gerrity, E., Keane, T.M. & Tuma, F. (eds), *The mental health consequences of torture*, Kluwer Academic/Plenum Publishers, Inc., New York, pp. 159–74.

Simpson, M.A. (1993) Traumatic stress and the bruising of the soul, In Wilson, J.P. & Raphael, B. (eds), *International Handbook of Traumatic Stress Syndromes*, Plenum Press, New York.

United Nations (1993) Security Council resolutions 808 (Feb. 22, 1993) and 827 (May 25 1993).

Victorian Foundation for Survivors of Torture (VFST) (1998) *Rebuilding Shattered Lives (Guide to those working with the survivors of torture and trauma)*, VFST, Melbourne.

Victorian Foundation for Survivors of Torture (VFST) (2002) *Rainbow Program—a school based program for refugee children and families*, VFST, Melbourne.

Victorian Health Promotion Foundation (2000) *Mental Health Promotion Plan. 1999–2002*, Foundation document, VicHealth, Melbourne.

8

Dichotomy or Decision Making: Specialisation and Mainstreaming in Health Service Design for Refugees

Cath Finney Lamb and Margaret Cunningham

Resettling refugees have special service needs that directly arise from experiences of deprivation and reduced access to health care. These occur in their home country, while fleeing their country, living for extended periods in refugee camp conditions, and when seeking asylum. Specific health service needs are also created by additional experiences of torture, or refugee trauma, including exposure to sexual violence. Health service literature and policy is peppered with debate about the relative merits of locating health care for special needs groups in specialised health care facilities or alternatively within mainstream health services. The articulation and development of this debate is important if health service planners are to ensure health services adequately meet these special needs.

This chapter proposes that the ability of various health service models to accommodate special service needs of refugees should be a key factor in the choice between specialised and mainstream health service models. Public health and human rights frameworks can be used to identify a set of generic special service needs for refugee and other marginalised groups. The chapter also describes factors that influence the capacity of specialised and mainstream services to provide the infrastructure support required for special needs.

Approaches to the choice of health service models for special needs groups

Following resettlement, refugee populations have special needs for clinical service delivery, interpersonal care and public health activities that may not always be common to mainstream populations. They may require specialist forms of clinical care to address the physical and mental health conditions produced by their refugee experience. Refugee clientele who have experienced trauma and human rights violations need interpersonal care that is trauma sensitive, and affirms their rights and dignity. Public health activities may also be required to address social conditions refugees experience during resettlement that produce health inequity, such as the lack of social networks and support, poverty and material deprivation, unemployment, and community prejudice.

Historically, health services in resettlement countries have adopted both specialised and mainstream health service models for refugee clientele groups. At the primary level of care, health care for newly arrived groups has been located in specialist refugee health care clinics (Harris & Telfer 2001; Hjern & Allebeck 1997; Shenson 1996) or located in mainstream primary care facilities (Fowler 1998; Hargreaves et al. 2000; Stanton et al. 2000). At the tertiary level of care, mental health care for survivors of torture and refugee trauma has been located in specialised torture and trauma centres (Allden 1998; Cunningham & Silove 1993). However, mental health care for refugees can also be provided through networks of mainstream mental health providers (Gray 1998) or in mainstream mental health facilities (Silove et al. 1997). These options present health service planners with a choice of service models that can be developed to meet refugee special needs.

A variety of mainstream and specialised service models are described that can accommodate special service needs for refugee and other marginalised groups. Mainstream health services provide health care for the bulk of the population. They can address special needs through tailoring service infrastructure to provide additional support, or by introducing targeted programs that address these needs. For example, services may tailor their organisational structures by employing personnel with specialised skills, such as client advocates or upskilled clinicians (Kelaher & Manderson 2000; Rosenheck 2000). Targeted programs may introduce clinics that provide comprehensive primary health care assessments (Fowler 1998) or conduct outreach programs (Goodburn 1994; McDonald 2001). In contrast, specialised health services are separated from mainstream services in order to provide service delivery for special needs groups such as those developed for indigenous communities, or specific women's health issues.

The adoption of a particular health service model for special needs groups is influenced by external factors such as existing health service infrastructures, and health and social policies. It can also be determined by political factors, historical events or prior health crises to which the health system has needed to respond (Ellencweig 1992). However, reactive/responsive modes of service development can lead to gaps in the system of care or make later strategic choices about changing health service models difficult. Systematic service planning can also be hindered by political factors, but nevertheless, it is needed to ensure effective population health care.

Systematic health service planning requires criteria on which to base decisions about service models. Health service planners traditionally make choices about the relative merits of various service models using an evidence-based approach addressing service outcomes, such as efficiency, equity, effectiveness, and sustainability (Mills & Ranson 2001; Reinke 2001). However, this planning information is often unavailable while health service models for new service contexts are being developed, because comparative health service evaluations can only be conducted after this has occurred. There is a paucity of published evaluations on services for refugees that is adequate to inform the decisions about which types of services will produce better outcomes.

There are supporters for both specialised, and mainstream approaches to refugee health care provision. Proponents on each side suggest that their approach is best because it will ensure refugees will not be excluded from appropriate health care. However, this simple dichotomy ignores the complexity of factors that contribute to the design of health services.

Proponents of mainstream health services argue that specialised services can produce health service ghettos, marginalise services from mainstream funding and policy support, and contribute to the exclusion of refugee clientele from mainstream services. Instead they advocate for mainstream services to accept responsibility for refugee health needs within their mandate (Wolmuth 1996). Proponents of specialised services argue that mainstream services cannot provide appropriate care for refugees. They advocate for specialised services to be developed to fill gaps in service provision, ensure health services are accessible to the clientele group, or provide the health service infrastructure to accommodate the special service delivery needs of clientele groups (Coventry et al. 2001; Silove et al. 1997; Weinstein et al. 2000).

An alternative to regarding the choice between mainstream and specialised services as a dichotomy is to recognise that these two types of service models support different types of service provision (Kelaher & Manderson 2000). This perspective leads to a variety of mainstream and specialised service options being adopted in service provision for populations with diverse needs (Kelaher & Manderson 2000). However, in order to make decisions about which service model will best meet client needs, health service planners need to identify which types of service provision are a priority for ensuring high quality, effective health care.

Special needs can represent immediate unmet needs for clinical and interpersonal care that directly impact on clientele health outcomes (Stanton et al. 2000; Weinstein et al. 2000; Wright et al. 1998), or service needs that are important for obtaining long-term outcomes. This is particularly recognised in clients with chronic conditions (Betz 1998; Rauen & Aubert 1992). Service delivery that accommodates special needs is therefore necessary for obtaining service outcomes. A primary factor in deciding which service models to adopt is the respective ability of the different service models to incorporate these special needs.

Using public health and human rights principles to identify special needs

Public health and human rights principles are useful for systematically identifying health service needs that may not be immediately provided by mainstream health services but which are important for achieving health outcomes. Public health and human rights frameworks for approaching health care also suggest some strategies and methods that health services can use to achieve these goals.

Public health principles emphasise that health services need to achieve health outcomes in population groups and define these outcomes in a holistic way: encompassing physical, mental, emotional, and spiritual dimensions of health (Baum 1998). These principles affirm health service goals that aim to redress health inequity and ensure optimal outcomes for unique clinical needs within minority groups, such as refugees (Baum 1998; Harris et al. 1999). Public health principles stress that health services need to address the determinants of health as well as treat disease in order to achieve health outcomes, and emphasise the importance of making health care relevant to its sociocultural context (Marmot 1999). They also recognise the need to arrange health services to respond to the social patterning of disease that occurs in specific population groups (Baum 1998). This includes recognising the need to provide clinical care for health conditions that are not common to the mainstream population.

Human rights principles emphasise certain ethical outcomes for health service provision. They assert that health services have a fundamental responsibility to uphold the human rights of clientele in clinical care and program delivery. Human rights frameworks for approaching health care advocate that service provision affirms the dignity of its clientele, upholds their rights to informed consent and decision making about their own health care, and ensures their rights to service access (Cunningham 2001). They affirm that health services have a responsibility to advocate for their client's rights in the community, particularly in situations where the denial of their human rights has a direct impact on their health (Alderslade 1995). This can occur in situations of individual discrimination, or when policies deny rights to health care or service access.

Public health and human rights principles should inform effective ways of conducting health services for the entire population. However, when applied to health service provision for marginalised groups, these principles can produce programs and models of service delivery that are distinct from the services of the mainstream population. These principles enable service delivery to be based on information on the social determinants that have been associated with disadvantaged health status (Lewis-Fernandez & Kleinman 1995; Shaw et al. 1999).

Clinicians operating within a holistic model of care may use holistic health care assessments to gauge social welfare, health care, and preventative health needs. This is typically followed up with client advocacy or referral (Conway-Welch et al. 1997; Lesser & Escoto-Lloyd 1999; Wright et al. 1998). For new refugee arrivals, this may mean helping to meet immediate settlement needs such as access to adequate housing, income and social welfare and health services (Baughan et al. 1990; Bowles 2001).

Several models of care address the sociocultural milieu in which personal and professional health care takes place. These can include holistic and sociocultural models of care. Within a clinical context, these health care models affirm the need to address sociocultural factors that impact on interpersonal care, such as bicultural communication, avoiding stereotypical communication approaches that may offend, accommodating cultural modes of decision making, and recognising traditional health care practices. Three particular factors that influence the sociocultural context of health care for refugees include refugee trauma, discrimination, and violations of human rights. Refugee clients have a particular need for trauma sensitive care that does not pathologise their trauma, nor retraumatise clients through simulating traumatic experiences (Bowles 2001; Stanton et al. 2000). As with other marginalised groups (Rosenheck 2000; Rosser et al. 1993), health care providers need to ensure that they provide non-judgemental care for refugees who have experienced stigma and discrimination in the community.

Health care models that uphold human rights seek to redress former human rights violations by ensuring the client's human rights in the clinical experience are explicit. Human rights within health care can be upheld through ensuring refugee clientele have the information required to make choices about their own health care and are empowered in making decisions about their self-care (Cunningham & Silove 1993). They can also adopt explicit value statements about clients' rights within their published service information.

Special programs that aim to improve access to health services for refugee groups recognise that social and cultural values can define or deny health care access, and uphold the clientele's rights to health care access. This can result in programs that aim to improve access to care such as the use of outreach workers and development of outreach programs; conducting community education about health services, or programs to strengthen community and agency referrals to health service agencies. Case management models and services brokers, such as bicultural workers, have been adopted to help refugee clients navigate the health system (Allden 1998; Kemp 1993).

Specialist forms of clinical care may be required in cases where rare diseases occur within a population group. Refugee groups in resettlement countries present a number of health conditions that arise from their refugee experience or country of origin (Ackerman 1997). Rare health conditions in refugee groups may be acute diseases, such as parasitic diseases (Walker & Jaranson 1999), or chronic conditions, such as mental health conditions related to refugee trauma (Silove et al. 1997). Health services need to respond with different types of health assessment at the primary level of care (Mollica 2001; Moreno et al. 2001; Weinstein et al. 2000), or the clinical management of rare diseases at a primary or tertiary level of care.

Decisions about which programs or models of service delivery to adopt for a particular clientele group will depend on the set of needs. For instance, clientele with primary care needs or chronic conditions requiring ongoing specialist care are likely to benefit most from holistic models of care. However, sociocultural models of care may be sufficient for client groups requiring specialty tertiary care for health conditions, such as infectious diseases or vitamin D deficiency. Similarly, programs that aim to improve health service access might address the needs of new arrivals for information about the health system, but address difficulties obtaining interpreters in small emerging communities.

Choosing specialised or mainstream services to meet special needs

Health service planners who aim to identify whether specialised and mainstream service models can adequately support a defined set of special service requirements need to undertake a relevant decision making and planning process. This section proposes that two issues need to be considered. Firstly, planners must determine the infrastructure support required for the special needs and identify whether specialised and/or mainstream services can provide this support. Secondly, they should consider whether it is feasible to reorientate mainstream services to provide the necessary support for special needs they may not immediately be able to provide.

Infrastructure support is foundational to ensuring special service needs can be accommodated within health services, because without this, service delivery cannot be sustained. Mainstream and specialised services differ in the infrastructure support they can offer. In some cases, both mainstream and specialised health services can provide sufficient service delivery support for clientele groups with special needs. In other cases, specialised services will more adequately provide support because they can specifically design their infrastructure to meet a defined set of special service requirements. Mainstream service models may be able to provide some additional resources or management support for special needs, and can make small modifications to organisational structures to accommodate them. However, when marginalised groups have a complex and comprehensive set of special needs, the pressure on mainstream services to provide infrastructure support can become too great.

An assessment of the infrastructure support required for a special needs group must define the support required for specific special needs as well as identify organisational and management structures required for general service delivery for the client group. For example, if primary health care services want to adopt holistic models of care, they may require additional resources to allow clinicians to conduct longer consultations (Harris & Knowlden 1999; Shorne et al. 2002). They may also be obliged to modify their organisational or management practices, by adopting specific forms of team structures or personnel management and support. Once the infrastructure requirements for supporting the special needs of a refugee clientele group have been identified, health service planners should identify which health service models best accommodate these needs. Since the health service literature for refugee populations in resettlement countries is primarily descriptive, there is little information to guide these decisions. However, lessons can be drawn from other marginalised groups with similar special needs.

Resources

Service delivery for special needs groups often requires more resources than would normally be required for similar service provision for the mainstream population. For example, health service access programs can require additional resources in order to modify bureaucratic barriers to care, such as complicated registration or inflexible scheduling (Gillis & Singer 1997; McQuistion et al. 1991). Refugee health service development often faces the problem of limited funding, particularly in the early stages of service development when needs are not recognised by mainstream funding arrangements. Within established services, locating and obtaining service funding from private donors, business, and industry has been used for service expansion, so that financial shortfalls do not decrease program delivery (Cunningham & Silove 1993; Mayer et al. 2001; McDaniel 1995). Specialised service structures can provide freedom from bureaucratic constraints that may limit fundraising being conducted (Aiken et al. 1997).

Expertise

Providing health care for refugees can involve some forms of expertise that are not common within mainstream services. Primary health care clinicians have been reported to provide inadequate health assessments for a variety of conditions that are common in refugees, including mental health, torture, or rare tropical diseases (Hargreaves et al. 2000; Thonneau et al. 1990; Weine et al. 2001; Weinstein et al. 2000). Holistic models of care can also require additional competencies in interpersonal care, client advocacy and networking. Specialised services can contribute to the development of expertise in a particular field through becoming Centres of Excellence. These types of services may have more flexibility to support research to inform the development of new clinical and treatment models and provide professional development to ensure staff are kept up to date with rapidly changing clinical knowledge (Kirmayer & Minas 2000; Poon et al. 1995; Rosser et al. 1993). This has occurred in torture and trauma service development, particularly in Australia (Cunningham & Silove 1993).

Organisational structures

Health services for refugees may need to organise team structures to include personnel with specialist expertise. Team structures that are designed to provide holistic care for refugee clientele groups can require a broad composition of skills. These teams are multi-disciplinary, and incorporate models for team communication and the division of roles and tasks that account for the impact that refugee trauma has on staff and team functioning (Bowles 2001). Specialised services may be more likely to adopt bicultural models in counselling (Silove et al. 1997), attract specialist skills (McDaniel 1995), and accommodate multi-disciplinary teams (Aiken et al. 1997).

Management

Managers should spend increased time in supporting service provision for special needs because of the increased volume of service activity that is associated with these clients. Refugee health services may be compelled to develop a wider range of interagency relationships than is normally required (Coventry et al 2001), in order to conduct advocacy, improve service access, or implement holistic models of care that require links to social welfare and human rights agencies. In these situations, managers will be required to spend time in developing additional organisational agreements, ensuring coordination mechanisms, and addressing political processes that ensures appropriate service coordination is maintained.

Managers should also ensure that internal policies and procedures are developed to support other special service activities for refugee groups. For example, refugee communities play an important role in referral and advice on appropriate care (Cunningham & Silove 1993; Keller et al. 1998). Management must ensure community members and clientele participate in health service planning through community consultations and representation on boards or committees (Conway-Welch et al. 1997; Cunningham & Silove 1993). Specialised services may allow greater flexibility in involving community members and organisations in their planning processes (Aiken et al. 1997).

Specific forms of personnel management are required for people working in refugee health. Professional support and management strategies are required to prevent burnout and vicarious trauma in refugee health staff. These can include the development of burnout prevention plans, development of team processes that manage team group dynamics in emotionally charged situations, training staff in personal care, and providing professional support through debriefing, team work, and managing staff workloads to contain work stressors (Catherall 1995; Yassen 1995). Organisational support provided in dedicated AID units has explained lower rates of burnout among staff when compared with mainstream services (Aiken et al. 1997). This suggests that specialised health services may have a greater capacity to provide organisational support to prevent burnout in refugee staff. Mainstream service providers who have refugee clientele as a small part of their caseload may not require management support, but may require links to specialised health services if support is required.

Reorientating mainstream services to meet special needs

Mainstream services are often the preferred option for service delivery for marginalised groups, even when specialised services can offer more support for special service needs. Mainstream services can provide services more efficiently for marginalised groups if they are geographically dispersed or too small to justify the expense of specialised health services. They may also be the only option for providing services for marginalised groups when health policies do not support the use of specialised services for minority groups, or when political conditions or economic reforms within the health system have limited existing specialised services which directly address their needs.

When mainstream services first start to work with marginalised groups, they can have a limited ability to support service delivery that addresses their special needs. However, capacity building programs can reorient the service infrastructure to more effectively meet these needs. Capacity building programs can aim to increase the expertise of mainstream personnel in providing specialist forms of clinical and interpersonal care. They can also endeavour to reorientate management practices to provide additional support for special service needs or introduce new organisational structures or programs to meet these needs.

There are a number of strategies that can be used to build the capacity of mainstream health services to meet special needs. Professional training programs and resources can increase the skills of mainstream service providers to provide appropriate clinical and interpersonal care for refugee health needs (Craft & Mulvey 2001; Cunningham & Silove 1993). Refugee health specialists can offer advice or consultancy to service managers who are undertaking service planning and development to more effectively meet refugee needs. At the middle management level, this type of planning can introduce an organisational mandate to meet refugee health needs and ensure coordination mechanisms are established between health services to provide continuity of care. Service planning initiatives can also result in changes to the organisational structure to provide services for the special needs groups in a new way.

The capacity of mainstream services to provide additional infrastructure support for special needs is also influenced by external factors within the health system, such as funding structures, health policy and professional training. Mainstream services can require more resources to meet the additional service burden introduced by clientele with special needs. However, resource allocation formulas may not recognise these needs (Kelaher & Manderson 2000). Resources may not be made available for special programs to be conducted within mainstream services that directly address special service needs. The inclusion of a refugee group's specific needs in mainstream health policies and plans is important for providing an organisational mandate to meet their needs. Health policies can be developed to provide a framework to guide mainstream services in integrating the special needs of marginalised groups into their service delivery and coordination between services (Coventry et al. 2001; Hargreaves et al. 2000). Professional education curricula influence the extent to which expertise is available within mainstream health services to provide refugee health care.

Programs that aim to reorientate the health system to meet special needs of refugees will therefore also need to modify factors within the health system that impact on the ability of mainstream services to meet these special needs. Refugee health specialists can work with professional training institutions to add competencies related to refugee health care into education curricula. They can also support professional education by lecturing students and supervising field placements (Wasylenki et al. 1997). Refugee health advocates can work with health service bureaucrats to reorientate funding structures to provide the additional resources needed to deliver services that address special needs. They can also work with health policy makers to redress policy gaps or develop specific health policies that provide frameworks for service development for refugee client groups.

Health service planners need to recognise that the mainstream service's capacity to provide infrastructure support for special needs will increase over time if capacity building initiatives are undertaken. Specialised services may be initially required to fill mainstream service gaps in meeting special needs. However, mainstream services may be able to effectively meet these needs after capacity building programs have been undertaken. Health service planners need to be able to make realistic assessments about the capacity of mainstream services to immediately accommodate special needs, and then how likely it is that they will be able to reorientate services to increase the available support. Factors that could be considered in each of these assessments are summarised in table 8.1.

Specialised services have a critical role in the capacity building for mainstream health services to meet refugee needs. Specialist resource units, such as the New South Wales Refugee Health Service, and specialised refugee health services, such as the torture and trauma services, can conduct interventions with health service providers and managers, and advocate for changes to policy, funding structure and professional education. Alternatively, networks of refugee health specialists such as the general practitioners or psychiatrists committed to human rights, can undertake advocacy and capacity building activities. Cooperative relationships with non-government organisations can highlight health impacts of

Table 8.1 Factors to consider in assessing the capacity of mainstream services to provide infrastructure support for special needs

Infrastructure support for special needs	Factors that influence the immediate capacity of mainstream services to meet special needs	Factors that influence the likelihood of mainstream health services being successfully reorientated to meet special needs
Expertise	Which of the required competencies are represented within mainstream services? Can additional competencies be taken up by mainstream service providers within the context of their daily work?	What are the barriers to expertise being taken up by mainstream providers? How much professional development for mainstream service providers needs to occur?
	Is there a need for specialist competencies to be developed within the context of service provision?	Can specialist expertise be integrated into mainstream education?
Resources	What additional resources are required to accommodate refugee special needs within mainstream services?	Can mainstream funding structures be reorientated to meet these needs?
	Do funding structures for mainstream services recognise the additional resources required to provide services to refugees?	What other additional sources of funding are available to supplement mainstream funding? What organisational structures are required to procure them?
Organisational and management support	How much additional organisational and management support is required to accommodate service needs within mainstream service structures?	Will the current organisational mandates, structures, and cultures within mainstream services enable change to occur?
	Can this additional support be easily integrated into mainstream service delivery?	What processes of organisational change will enable the adoption of service functions to meet special needs? How long will organisational change take to occur?
	Do health policies exist that provide guidance for service provision for refugee groups?	Can policy be developed to facilitate the integration of special service needs for refugees into mainstream service delivery? E.g. Support for professional training and development. Best practice guidelines.

social policies. International and federal policy advisory bodies also have an important role to play, particularly if the special needs group has been identified in policy frameworks. Thus, there will always be a need for some specialised services to retain specialist knowledge about service delivery for refugee groups.

Conclusion

Lessons from other marginalised groups demonstrate that the evolution of specialised and mainstream models of care can reflect migration policies and ideologies, rather than need (Kelaher & Manderson 2000; Kirmayer & Minas 2000; Kunitz & Brady 1995). In addition, debates about the use of specialised and mainstream health services for marginalised groups often reflect broader public debates about service provision for these groups. In resettlement countries, the political environment is becoming increasingly sensitive to the costs of refugee settlement. Refugee health advocates need to ensure that decision making about health service provision for refugees will protect their human rights for health care.

Acknowledgments

The authors acknowledge Professor Anthony Zwi, who proposed that this chapter focus on examining arguments for the use of specialised or mainstream health service structures for refugees, using the health service literature from other marginalised groups. We would also like to thank Dr Mitchell Smith, who commented on numerous drafts of this chapter and Aaron Silver, who aided with the literature search and collection of journal articles that informed this chapter.

Recommended reading

Ackerman, L.K .(1997) Health problems of refugees, *Journal of the American Board of Practice*, 10(5): 337–48.

Bowles, R. (2001) Social work with refugee survivors of torture and trauma, In Alston, M. & McKinnon, J. (eds), *Social work. Fields of practice*, Oxford University Press, Melbourne.

Fowler, N. (1998) Providing primary health care to immigrants and refugees: the North Hamilton experience, *Canadian Medical Association Journal*, 159(4): 388–91.

Kemp, C. (1993) Health services for refugees in countries of second asylum, *International Nursing Review*, 40(1): 21–4.

Mann, J., Gruskin, S., Grodin, M.L. & Annas, G.J. (eds) (1999) *Health and Human Rights: A Reader*, Routledge, New York.
Mollica, R.F. (2001) Assessment of trauma in primary care, *Journal of the American Medical Association*, 285(9): 1213.

References

Ackerman, L.K. (1997) Health problems of refugees, *Journal of the American Board of Practice*, 10(5): 337–48.
Aiken, L.H., Sloane, D.M. & Lake, E.T. (1997) Satisfaction with inpatient acquired immunodeficiency syndrome care, A national comparison of dedicated and scattered-based units, *Medical Care*, 35(9): 948–62.
Alderslade, R. (1995) Human rights and medical practice, including reference to the joint Oslo statements of September 1993 and March 1994, *Journal of Public Health Medicine*, 17(3): 335–42.
Allden, K. (1998) The Indochinese Psychiatry Clinic: trauma and refugee mental health treatment in the 1990s, *Journal of Ambulatory Care Management*, 21(2): 30–8.
Baughan, D.M., White-Baughan, J., Pickwell, S., Bartlome, J. & Wong, S. (1990) Primary care needs of Cambodian refugees, *Journal of Family Practice*, 30(5): 565–8.
Baum, F. (1998) *The new public health: An Australian perspective*, Oxford University Press, Melbourne.
Betz, C. (1998) Facilitating the transition of adolescents with chronic conditions from pediatric to adult health care and community settings, *Issues in Comprehensive Pediatric Nursing*, 21: 97–115.
Bowles, R. (2001) Social work with refugee survivors of torture and trauma, In eds, Alston, M. & McKinnon, J. (ed) *Social work. Fields of practice*, Oxford University Press, Melbourne.
Catherall, D.R. (1995) Preventing institutional secondary traumatic stress disorder, In Figley, C.R. (ed.), *Compassion Fatigue*, Brummar Mazel, New York.
Conway-Welch, C., Fogel, C., Holm, K., Killien, M., Marion, L., McBride, A., Shaver, J., Simms, L., Swanson, K., Taylor, D. & Woods, N. (1997) Women's Health and Women's Health Care: Recommendations of the 1996 AAN Expert panel on Women's Health, *Nursing Outlook*, 45: 7–15.
Coventry, L., Guerra, D., MacKenzie, C., & Pinkey, S. (2001) *Wealth of All Nations: identification of strategies to assist refugee young people in transition to independence—a report to the National Youth Affairs Research Scheme 2001*, Centre for Multicultural Youth Issues, Melbourne
Craft, E.M. & Mulvey, K.P. (2001) Addressing lesbian, gay, bisexual and transgender issues from the inside: One Federal Agency's approach, *American Journal of Public Health*, 91(6): 889–91.
Cunningham M., Fielding A. (2001) Linking human rights practice in health care to refugees: Challenges for health care and refugee service providers, International Conference 'UN Convention: *Where to From Here*', UNSW, December.
Cunningham, M. & Silove, D. (1993) Principles of treatment and service development for torture and trauma survivors, In Wilson, J.P. & Raphael, B. (eds), *International Handbook of Traumatic Stress Syndromes*, Plenum Press, New York, pp. 751–62.
Ellencweig, A.Y. (1992) *Analysing health systems: a modular approach*, Oxford Medical Press, Oxford.

Fowler, N. (1998) Providing primary health care to immigrants and refugees: the North Hamilton experience, *Canadian Medical Association Journal*, 159(4): 388–91.

Gillis, L.M. & Singer, J. (1997) Breaking through the barriers: healthcare for the homeless, *Journal of Nursing Adminstration*, 27(6): 30–4.

Goodburn, A. (1994) A place of greater safety, *Nursing Times*, 90(28): 46–8.

Gray, G. (1998) Treatment of survivors of political torture: administrative and clinical issues, *Journal of Ambulatory Care Management*, 21(2): 39-42; discussion 43–55.

Hargreaves, S., Holmes, A. & Friedland, J.S. (2000) Refugees, asylum seekers, and general practice: room for improvement? *British Journal of General Practice*, 50(456): 531–2.

Harris, E., Nutbeam, D., Sainsbury, P., King, L. & Whitecross, P. (1999) Finding a way forward, (ed.) *Perspectives on health inequity*, Australian Centre for Health Promotion, Sydney.

Harris, M. & Knowlden, S. (1999) Clinical perspective: A general practitioner response to health differentials, In Harris, E., Sainsbury, P. & Nutbeam, D. (eds), *Perspectives on Health Inequity*, the Australian Centre for Health Promotion, Sydney.

Harris, M.F. & Telfer, B.L. (2001) The health needs of asylum seekers living in the community, *Medical Journal of Australia*, 175: 589–93.

Hjern, A. & Allebeck, P. (1997) Health examinations and health services for asylum seekers in Sweden, *Scandinavian Journal of Social Medicine*, 25(3): 207–9.

Kelahcr, M. & Manderson, L. (2000) Migration and mainstreaming: matching health services to immigrants' needs in Australia, *Health Policy*, 54(1): 1–11.

Keller, A.S., Saul, J.M. & Eisenman, D.P. (1998) Caring for survivors of torture in an urban, municipal hospital, *Journal of Ambulatory Care Management*, 21(2): 20–9.

Kemp, C. (1993) Health services for refugees in countries of second asylum, *International Nursing Review*, 40(1): 21–4.

Kirmayer, L.J. & Minas, H. (2000) The future of cultural psychiatry: an international perspective, *Canadian Journal of Psychiatry*, 45(5): 438–46.

Kunitz, S.J. & Brady, M. (1995) Health care policy for Aboriginal Australians: the relevance of the American Indian experience, *Australia and New Zealand Journal of Public Health*, 19(6): 549–58.

Lesser, J. & Escoto-Lloyd, S. (1999) Health-related problems in a vulnerable population: pregnant teens and adolescent mothers, *Nursing Clinics of North America*, 34(2): 289–99.

Lewis-Fernandez, R. & Kleinman, A. (1995) Cultural psychiatry. Theoretical, clinical, and research issues *Psychiatric Clinics of North America*, 18(3): 433–48.

Marmot, M. (1999) Introduction, In Marmot, M. & Wilkinson, R.G. (ed) *Social Determinants of Health*, Oxford University Press, New York.

Mayer, K., Applebaum, J., Rogers, T., & Lo, W. (2001) The evolution of the Fenway Community Health model, *American Journal of Public Health*, 91(6): 892–96.

McDaniel, J.S. (1995) Compassionate mental health care for persons with HIV and AIDS, *Psychiatr Serv*, 46(10): 1061–4.

McDonald, A. (2001) Sanctuary in Glasgow, *Community Practitioner*, 74(3): 86–7.

McQuistion, H.L., D'Ercole, A. & Kopelson, E. (1991) Urban Street Outreach: Using clinical principles to steer the system, *New Directions for Mental Health Services*, 52: 17–27.

Mills, A. & Ranson, M.K. (2001) The design of health systems, In Merson, M.H., Black, R.E. & Mills, A.J. (eds), *International Public Health. Diseases, Programs, Systems and Policies*, Aspen Publishers Inc., Gaithersburg, Maryland.

Mollica, R.F. (2001) Journal of the American Medical Association: assessment of trauma in primary care, *Journal of the American Medical Association*, 285(9): 1213.

Moreno, A., Piwowarczyk, L. & Grodin, M.A. (2001) Journal of the American Medical Association: human rights violations and refugee health, *Journal of the American Medical Association*, 285(9): 1215.

Poon, M.-C., Israels, S.J. & Lillicrap, D.P. (1995) Hemophilia and von Willebrand's disease: 1. Diagnosis, comprehensive care and assessment, *Canadian Medical Association Journal*, 153(1): 19–25.

Rauen, K.K. & Aubert, E.J. (1992) A brighter future for adults who have Myelomeningocele—one form of spina bifida, *Orthopaedic Nursing*, 11(3): 16–26.

Reinke, W.A. (2001) Health systems management, In Merson, M.H., Black, R.E. & Mills, A.J. (eds), *International Public Health. Diseases, Programs, Systems and Policies*, Aspen Publishers Gaithesburg, Maryland.

Rosenheck, R. (2000) Primary care satellite clinics and improved access to general and mental health services, *Health Services Research*, 35(4): 777–90.

Rosser, B.R.S., Coleman, E. & Ohmans, P. (1993) Safer sex maintenance and reduction of unsafe sex among homosexually active men: a new therapeutic approach, *Health Education Research*, 8(1): 19–34.

Shaw, M., Dorling, D. & Davey Smith, G. (1999) Poverty, social exclusion, and minorities, In Marmot, M. & Wilkinson, R.G. (eds), *Social Determinants of Health*, Oxford University Press, Oxford, pp. 211–39.

Shenson, D. (1996) A primary care clinic for the documentation and treatment of human rights abuses, *Journal of General Internal Medicine*, 11(9): 533–8.

Shorne, L., McCaul, M. & Gunn, J. (2002) 'Beam me up Scotty': trekking from women's health to General Practice, *New Doctor*, 76: 22–5.

Silove, D., Manicavasagar, V., Beltran, R., Le, G., Nguyen, H., Phan, T. & Blaszczynski, A. (1997) Satisfaction of Vietnamese patients and their families with refugee and mainstream mental health services, *Psychiatric Services*, 48(8): 1064–9.

Stanton, J., Kaplan, I. & Webster, K. (2000), Role of Australian doctors in refugee health care, *Current Therapeutics*, December 1999–January 2000: 24–8.

Thonneau, P., Gratton, J. & Desrosiers, G. (1990) Health profile of applicants for refugee status (admitted into Quebec between August 1985 and April 1986), *Canadian Journal of Public Health*, 81(3): 182–6.

Walker, P.F. & Jaranson, J. (1999) Refugee and immigrant health care, *Medical Clinics of North America*, 83(4): 1103–20.

Wasylenki, D.A., Cohen, C.A. & McRobb, B.R. (1997) Creating community agency placments for undergraduate medical education: a program description, *Canadian Medical Association Journal*, 156(3): 379–83.

Weine, S.M., Kuc, G., Dzudza, E., Razzano, L. & Pavkovic, I. (2001) PTSD among Bosnian refugees: a survey of providers' knowledge, attitudes and service patterns, *Community Mental Health Journal*, 37(3): 261–71.

Weinstein, H.M., Sarnoff, R.H., Gladstone, E. & Lipson, J.G. (2000) Physical and psychological health issues of resettled refugees in the United States, *Journal of Refugee Studies*, 13(3): 303–27.

Wolmuth, P. (1996) Removing the barriers, *Health Visitor*, 69(3): 93–4.

Wright, E.R., Gonzalez, B.A., Werner, J.A., Laughner, S.T. & Wallace, M. (1998) Indiana Youth Access Project, a model for responding to HIV risk behaviours of gay, lesbian and the bisexual youth in the Heartland, *Society for Adolescent Medicine*, 23(25): 83–95.

Yassen, J. (1995.) Preventing secondary traumatic stress disorder, In Figley, C.R. (ed.) *Compassion Fatigue*, Brummar Mazel, New York.

9

Operation Safe Haven: Health Service Delivery to Temporary Evacuees

Mitchell Smith and Bronwen Harvey

Introduction

In early 1999 there was a marked escalation in the conflict between opposing forces in the former Yugoslav republic of Kosovo. This culminated in so-called 'ethnic cleansing' of residents of ethnic Albanian origin, and the flight of refugees into neighbouring countries. When NATO forces commenced bombing, many more thousands of Albanian Kosovars fled into Albania and the former Yugoslav Republic of Macedonia.

When the capacity of those two countries to cope with the influx was exceeded, the United Nations High Commissioner for Refugees (UNHCR) sought to relocate some of the refugees in a number of countries, including Australia. In early April 1999 Australia agreed to provide temporary safe haven to 4000 people. The UNHCR request was subsequently put on hold for several weeks in the hope solutions could be found in countries closer to Kosovo. The request was reactivated on 1 May 1999 as the flood of refugees continued to exceed available capacity in the region.

The evacuation, known in Australia as Operation Safe Haven, saw the first Kosovar Albanian evacuees arrive on Australian soil on 7 May, only six days after the final decision was made to proceed (Department of Immigration and Multicultural and Indigenous Affairs 1999b). A total of 19 chartered and commercial flights brought evacuees at intervals of three to five days over a period of six weeks, with the final group arriving in Australia on 23 June 1999.

In August of the same year, violence erupted in East Timor preceding the referendum on independence from Indonesia, and increased following the vote on 30 August. Staff of the United Nations Mission in East

Timor (UNAMET) were at risk, as were their families and hundreds of locals who had sought shelter in the UNAMET compound in Dili. At the request of the UN, Australia agreed to evacuate 1800 people from the compound by air to Darwin, and formally announced the initiative on 6 September. The airlift commenced in the ensuing days and was completed by 14 September 1999.

This chapter describes the response of health services in Australia to these emergencies. It presents an overview of the planning and implementation of health service delivery throughout Operation Safe Haven and discusses some of the lessons learnt.

The Kosovar operation

Operation Safe Haven had no precedent in Australia. The short time frames involved were problematic for all agencies in terms of planning and implementation, particularly where funding arrangements had to be negotiated (DIMIA 1999b). Uncertainty regarding dates and times of arrivals, departures, and other key events was a theme that continued throughout the operation. Despite these and other challenges, the response on the ground was generally successful, and one that reflected the experience of agencies in Australia in delivering services in a context of cultural and linguistic diversity (DIMIA 1999a).

The Australian Government's compliance with the UNHCR request for *temporary* relocation established the overarching parameters for Operation Safe Haven. Evacuees were not eligible to apply for permanent asylum in Australia and were to be repatriated back to Kosovo as soon as UNHCR determined it was safe to do so. The initial duration of the safe haven visas was three months, but was later extended.

Accommodation was provided on military bases, known as Haven Centres, throughout the evacuees' stay. This decision raised some concern among health workers because of the potential for continued trauma to people fleeing a conflict situation. Eight current or former military sites across five states were selected, based on the numbers to be accommodated, the capacity to prepare the sites within the time frame of the evacuation, and the need for minimal impact on normal Australian Defence Force activities. Proximity to support services, including medical ones, was a secondary consideration and the location of sites had subsequent impacts on how services were provided (Coombe 2000; Roper 1999). The evacuees were free to move around Australia. However, provision was made for services and financial support to be available only to those who remained on the bases.

A Commonwealth Government Interdepartmental Committee, the Kosovo Task Force, was established to coordinate the planning and implementation of Operation Safe Haven. The task force was headed by the Department of Immigration and Multicultural and Indigenous Affairs (DIMIA). The other lead agencies were the Department of Defence (DOD) and the Department of Health and Aged Care (DHAC), supported by Emergency Management Australia (EMA) and Health Services Australia (HSA). This latter agency is normally contracted by DIMIA to undertake health assessments for people making onshore visa applications. A range of other agencies was also represented on the task force.

The role of the DHAC was to advise DIMIA, define roles and responsibilities for screening and health care during the reception and safe haven phases, develop health care protocols with the states and territories, and work with local health authorities regarding follow-up processes (DHAC 1999). DHAC also provided funding for Health Services Australia, state health authorities, and torture and trauma counselling services. A further role was liaison with UNHCR, the International Organisation for Migration, DIMIA, and state health departments regarding repatriation issues.

Health screening of the evacuees was a Commonwealth requirement to ensure Australian public health and safety, and early identification and treatment of any serious conditions. This led to the decision to incorporate a reception centre phase during which evacuees received comprehensive health assessments and any immediately necessary treatment, prior to being transported to their haven centres. Health Services Australia (HSA) undertook the initial health screenings, both in Macedonia prior to embarkation and in Sydney during the reception phase. HSA staff also accompanied each flight.

State emergency management plans were activated in several instances (Bayman et al. 2000; DIMIA 1999a). These plans, developed to address internal disasters, were not optimal for addressing Operation Safe Haven issues. For example, the roles of the torture and trauma counselling services, crucial to the evacuees, were unclear within the disaster plan frameworks. However, activation of such plans provided the intended benefits of easier mobilisation of resources and the involvement of additional agencies with experience in disaster recovery.

Committees involving relevant state and local area health authorities addressed health planning issues locally. These committees worked to the protocols developed by the funding agency (DHAC), but adapted them to local conditions.

Health screening and health service protocols

Some limited data were available on the health status of Kosovars prior to the conflict and on health problems detected among the Kosovars in camps in Albania (Public Health Laboratory Service (PHLS) 1999). However, the lack of detail made the development of health screening and health service protocols difficult. Of the communicable diseases, tuberculosis (TB) was known to be at moderate levels (around 40 per 100,000) but increasing in response to refugee stress and interruption of treatment; hepatitis A was highly endemic; hepatitis B 'moderate to high'; HIV was low. Immunisation rates had been falling, with children born after April 1998 likely to have never been vaccinated. Pregnancy rates were high. In the camps in Europe there had been no outbreaks of infectious diseases, although sporadic cases of gastrointestinal and respiratory infections and a few cases of viral meningitis had been reported. Over half of consultations in the camps had been for chronic diseases including diabetes, hypertension, and asthma. The UN had commenced a basic immunisation program for 0 to 5 year olds.

Australian immigration legislation requires that permanent immigrants and some long-stay visitors have a full medical examination, including chest X-ray screening for TB and HIV screening (for those aged 16 years or older and 15 years or older, respectively) prior to being issued a visa to enter the country. However, given the short time frames and limited facilities available, the task force decided to limit the scope of pre-embarkation medical examinations in Macedonia to a 'fitness to fly' check, with full screening delayed until arrival in Australia. The pre-embarkation check thus focused on ensuring the ability to endure the long air flight and associated ground travel, and on excluding anyone with active TB or other communicable condition. Women over thirty-six weeks gestation were also excluded from flying.

A number of health issues presented during transit from Macedonia. Hyperactivity and vomiting among children on early flights was linked to an excess of caffeinated and carbonated drinks. These problems reduced on later flights when the intake of such drinks was limited [Health Services Australia, pers. comm.]. Other problems in-flight were more serious. On the sixth flight, health staff encountered two young children with high fever of unknown cause raising concerns about possible meningitis. Other incidents included a woman with an anaphylactoid reaction due to aspirin and a young woman who collapsed and appeared hypoglycaemic

(Health Services Australia 1999a). These cases highlighted the need to ensure accompanying doctors were comfortable working with seriously ill cases in a confined space with minimal back-up and no possibility of transferring cases out [Health Services Australia, pers. comm.].

The most common problems on arrival at the reception centre in Sydney were fatigue, travel sickness from the airport bus trip, and ear barotrauma from what was, for most, their first experience of flying. Advice about these problems was fed back to HSA, with reduction in the incidence among evacuees on later flights.

The focus of the health screening conducted on arrival in Australia was to identify immediate and short-term health needs and to protect public health. The only relevant health screening protocol available in Australia in 1999 had been designed for screening of Vietnamese boat people in the 1980s (National Health and Medical Research Council (NHMRC) 1995). This protocol was rapidly modified in consultation with the Communicable Diseases Network Australia and New Zealand (CDNANZ) and revised as further information became available.

All evacuees were required to give a medical history and undergo clinical examination, including blood pressure and assessment of mental state. Those aged 16 years and above had a chest X-ray, and urinalysis was done for those over 5 years. HIV testing was not performed given the temporary nature of the evacuees' stay. Apart from antenatal screening of pregnant women, no other routine tests were done. Dental assessment was offered on a voluntary basis. In view of the short turnaround times, it was decided to delay immunisation until after transfer to the haven centres interstate. Detailed protocols for TB screening and follow-up and for dental assessment and treatment were developed. Over the six-week reception period, HSA performed over 3900 health checks and 2500 X-rays, of which 309 were flagged for follow-up (Health Services Australia 1999b).

The transfer of medical information to the haven centres was essential to ensure problems identified during screening were monitored and treatment commenced. Initially, however, there was no agreed process for information transfer. While a number of databases were created to record the details of TB patients and other public health findings, these were for case management and surveillance purposes respectively (Bennett et al. 2000). A database for patients needing follow-up was attempted but not sustained, as staffing levels during the hectic reception phase were limited. Moreover some haven centres could not access the database information due to a lack of matching software. Medical records were generally photocopied and transferred as hard copy, but records often arrived some time after the group and, in one case, not at all.

Given the anticipated stay of three to six months, health authorities were asked to provide evacuees with medical and dental care focused on conditions requiring management in the immediate or short term. A number of interventions were excluded from the standard protocol. These included complex, staged surgical treatments, circumcision, tubal ligation or vasectomy, surgical investigations for infertility and complex infertility treatments. Immunisation was offered to children and adults in accordance with the Australian Vaccination Schedule current at that time (National Health and Medical Research Council 2000). Health promotion activities, such as information about the hazards of smoking, were included but mass screening of asymptomatic evacuees for breast, cervical, and other cancers was not. Specific provision was made for torture and trauma counselling and for the provision of mental health services.

On repatriation, evacuees were to be provided with a personal health status summary detailing the treatments they had received in Australia and their current health status and medications. Sufficient medications were provided to complete short-term treatments, including TB therapy, and to enable three months' treatment of long-term conditions.

A national protocol was developed for immunisation for staff and volunteers working in the reception and haven centres. The requirement was for immunisations to be up-to-date in accordance with the NHMRC recommendations (National Health and Medical Research Council 2000) for each occupational group. No additional vaccines were recommended. Pregnant women were advised to be aware of their rubella and chicken pox immunity status.

Agency staff and volunteers concerned about health risks from working in the haven centres were provided with relevant information based on the national protocol. In New South Wales a document was prepared with advice about the level and nature of risks for exposure to infectious diseases. The potential for psychological impacts on staff and volunteers from working with traumatised people was also addressed (Smith 1999).

Health services model

All haven centres adopted an integrated primary care based model, which resulted in most primary care and some specialist/consultant care being provided on site. Services established at the centres on either a sessional or full-time basis included: public and environmental health; general practice; nursing; maternal and child health; immunisation; mental health; torture and trauma counselling; and dental health (Ali et al. 1999; Carrello et al. 2000; Department of Human Services South Australia 1999; Murphy undated; Roper 1999; South Western Sydney Area Health Service 2000).

Some centres provided allied health services such as physiotherapy and optometry on-site (Ali et al. 1999; Merriman 1999). Specialist clinics (e.g. antenatal, gynaecological, TB/respiratory, paediatric) were established on-site at some centres, while at others these services were accessed through local hospital outpatient clinics or private rooms. Whether or not services were provided on-site was generally related to the distance from the centres to secondary and tertiary services.

Centres established basic in-patient facilities to enable patients to be observed overnight or for a period during the day. These facilities reduced the number of cases referred to hospital, minimised family separations and reduced the logistic challenges of transport and sharing of interpreters with the hospital (National Public Health Partnership 1999; South Western Sydney Area Health Service 2000). When necessary, hospital admissions were generally arranged at the nearest public hospital with appropriate facilities.

Different states utilised the private health sector to varying degrees. Western Australia (WA), in particular, utilised private providers, often being able to negotiate free or reduced-fee services (Carrello et al. 2000). In New South Wales private providers were only used when the patient chose to pay or special agreement was reached with the Commonwealth.

Interpreter service provision was key and was a challenge for health and other service providers nationally, given the limited number of accredited Albanian-speaking interpreters.

Torture and trauma/mental health services

Australia has a national network of services to work specifically with migrants who are survivors of torture and/or refugee trauma. These services were contracted by the Commonwealth Government to provide counselling and other relevant activities during Operation Safe Haven. In some sites the torture and trauma (T&T) services remained quite distinct in location and role from other health services, while at others they worked side by side with mental health staff (Merriman 1999).

Given the acutely traumatised population and the temporary nature of the haven in Australia, the T&T network adapted its normal approach, while maintaining a combination of community, group, and individually targeted strategies (Stow & Leary undated). An informal, community-based approach was found to be most useful, particularly as many Kosovars resisted one-to-one counselling as a mode of therapy.

In Victoria the main aims of the T&T service were: to increase perceptions of safety, meaning to life and dignity; to normalise attachments; and to reduce fear. Group work, initially, had limited success with low attendances and was subsequently reorientated to create special interest groups, such as fishing. At a number of haven centres, the classrooms on-site became locations for group work opportunities (Department of Human Services South Australia 1999; Stow & Leary undated). In WA, the aim was to provide a 'safe environment for normalisation of psychological response to trauma' (Carrello et al. 2000). This was done through a combination of community approaches and self-help strategies for their time in the haven and for their eventual return, and involved a range of projects.

Staff training and education was an important role of the T&T services, helping to prepare staff and volunteers from health and other agencies for work with a traumatised population. Regular, ongoing information sessions throughout the project were considered beneficial (Trauma Counselling Support Service undated). Formal and informal debriefing and counselling of staff from health and other agencies was a role shared by all of the T&T services. Demands for this increased towards the end of the project, as staff tried to come to terms with the uncertainty and sadness about evacuees being repatriated (Trauma Counselling Support Service undated). Debriefings for interpreters were particularly important as they were constantly exposed to traumatic stories from the residents, with whom they formed close bonds. At times there were significant concerns for the well-being of the interpreter staff.

Volunteers were used to assist the work of the T&T services in some havens, with mixed success. While the use of volunteers sourced from the Kosovar residents and the external community had some benefits, it also presented challenges (Ali et al. 1999; Trauma Counselling Support Service undated). This included difficulties in restricting volunteers to appropriate role limits, and perceptions that volunteers from the haven community were receiving favourable treatment.

Other services contributed greatly to the psychological health and well-being of the evacuees. Child and youth health teams and mental health staff were variously involved (Department of Human Services South Australia 1999; Merriman 1999). Education providers, child playgroup staff, recreational services, and religious bodies were some of the most important contributors to a positive outlook for haven residents.

Health staffing

Staff planning was difficult for a number of reasons. The level of health service demand was initially unknown and the duration of stay uncertain. Operation Safe Haven work was additional to normal work demands for most health staff. In the early stages, staff were part-time and/or short stay, which was not ideal for continuity and interaction with the residents (Trauma Counselling Support Service undated). Some service needs were unforeseen in initial planning and had to be addressed later.

A shortage of nurses at local hospitals required the frequent use of agency nursing staff. Administration and medical record staff were generally seconded from local hospitals and health services to work on-site. The staffing of T&T counselling services was particularly difficult, given the limited number of trained counsellors available and the need to maintain normal services elsewhere. Initial funding uncertainties delayed the employment of staff in some cases.

Local divisions of general practice played key roles in providing general practitioners (GPs) (Carrello et al. 2000; DIMIA 1999a; South Western Sydney Area Health Service 2000). Different selection processes were used for GPs in different states. For example, in WA doctors were selected against specific criteria, while in New South Wales all interested GPs were included in the roster. South Australia opted to use doctors employed already in the Migrant Health Service, Community Health Centres and a Travellers' Medical Centre (Department of Human Services South Australia 1999).

The primary care model worked well, although professional staff often had to work outside their normal roles. For example, at some sites nurses were challenged by having greater autonomy than in a standard hospital or community setting, operating more like nurse practitioners (Ali et al. 1999; Department of Human Services South Australia 1999; South Western Sydney Area Health Service 2000).

Specific health issues

Smoking rates were very high, particularly among men. This created difficulties on the long (smoke-free) flights from Europe. Initial cigarette distribution, performed as a 'humanitarian' gesture in some states, was ceased for health promotion reasons, and this had an impact on the psychological status of some residents (Trauma Counselling Support Service undated). Sugar intake was very high, especially in children, reflected by a high level of dental caries. Cultural differences in parenting techniques and attitudes to domestic violence and punishment of children presented challenges to staff and required sensitive handling (Coombe 2000).

At the haven primary care clinic in Sydney, the mean consultation rate was just over four visits per patient over a six-month period. The top five diagnoses were upper respiratory infection, disease of the teeth or gums, lower respiratory infection, headache, and otitis media (Smith et al. 2001).

Overt psychological presentations to the clinic were low in prevalence, a finding among Kosovar evacuees to the United Kingdom (UK) as well (Bowie 1999). Further common reasons for presentation at other haven clinics included skin conditions, musculoskeletal problems, diabetes, hypertension, gastric disorders, and renal disease (Ali et al. 1999; Carrello et al. 2000). Other problems recorded by havens included head lice, chicken pox, bronchiolitis, a few cases of hepatitis A, iron deficiency anaemia, and several inguinal hernias. Rarer conditions included a number of cancers and thyroid disease. Although national data on the occurrence of various conditions was not collated, the spectrum of disease seen was not considered unusual for the size and demographics of the population. Twenty-five Kosovars aged from 2 years to 65 years were commenced on treatment for proven or suspected tuberculosis. Eight of these were confirmed through bacteriological culture, giving a prevalence rate of confirmed cases of approximately 200 per 100,000 (Smith et al. 2001).

The Australian findings were consistent with those in other countries. A report on health care for 4000 Kosovars who were accepted as refugees for resettlement in the USA found them to be generally in good health. The TB prevalence was 148 per 100,000 (culture confirmed). Head lice were prominent. In a ten-week period approximately 1000 dental visits were recorded (Centers for Disease Control and Prevention 1999).

Repatriation

'Voluntary' repatriation of Kosovars from Australia began in early July 1999. In August the Commonwealth Government offered those who returned before the end of October 1999 a 'winter reconstruction allowance' of $3000 per adult and $500 for each child under 18 years of age. This was to assist the Kosovars in rebuilding their homes and livelihoods. Many nevertheless remained until late in the year, with a small number of medical cases still present 12 months after their arrival.

The return to Kosovo presented a new aspect to the operation. A number of Kosovars were keen to return as soon as feasible to seek out family members or to ensure land and houses were not lost to others. Some left without completing medical treatment. Others left without necessary medication, either by choice or due to delayed communication of return dates. A number of haven residents were frightened of returning to their homeland, fearing for their safety there. This had an impact on staff caring for the evacuees.

Larger repatriations often presented logistic difficulties, with limited time available to arrange medications, discharge reports and copies of results (South Western Sydney Area Health Service 2000). In addition, anyone under active medical treatment needed a review to determine fitness to return. Where possible, persons on TB treatment were kept in Australia until the completion of treatment, as medications and appropriate monitoring could not be guaranteed in Kosovo.

The East Timorese operation

The arrival of evacuees from East Timor came while the Kosovar safe haven operation was still underway. Valuable lessons learnt were applied to this second group of short-term emergency arrivals. Two Emergency Response Plans were implemented to assist with the evacuation and arrival of East Timorese from the United Nations Mission in East Timor (UNAMET) compound in Dili and arrival in Darwin. One was the national COMRECEPLAN that normally focuses on Australian citizens requiring evacuation from overseas. The other was the local Northern Territory Counter-Disaster Plan. Under these plans Territory Health Services (THS) had joint responsibility for health and welfare services (McComb 2001).

As with the Kosovars, a large range of agencies was involved in providing services. Non-governmental organisations, a number of which had disaster management experience from past floods in the region, played an important role. The importance of the Catholic Church was recognised very early, given the strong faith among many East Timorese.

The East Timorese were accommodated in a tent city at the Kalymnian Centre, which had been set up through the joint efforts of a number of government departments and the local Greek community. This was a temporary measure pending transfer to haven centres around the country, as for the Kosovar evacuees.

The THS responsibilities included: health triage and screening; advice on persons 'fit to fly' interstate; control of infectious diseases; welfare, medical, hospital and public health services; and overseeing essential hospitality services such as meals, bedding, and clothing. THS staff were invited to be involved either as part of their work or on a volunteer basis. Community health nurses from a number of outlying centres, experienced in remote and indigenous health, contributed. The local Division of General Practice was also a key partner with over 100 doctors willing to offer their services on a roster basis, supporting salaried THS medical officers (McComb 2001).

Health screening protocols and health service delivery

The protocols used for the Kosovars were reviewed and adapted to take account of the different disease risks in the East Timorese population. The high burden of tuberculosis was recognised early and the age for chest X-ray screening was reduced to 12 years. Malaria screening for pregnant women and anyone presenting with a fever was introduced. Blanket treatment for gut parasites for all people over 6 months of age was recommended as was the routine administration of vitamin A to children up to 12 years of age after arrival at the safe haven or earlier if ill or malnourished.

Service delivery followed the model used for the Kosovar Operation Safe Haven. Staff in the havens receiving East Timorese found that the previous experience assisted planning and implementation for the new arrivals (Carrello et al. 2000; South Western Sydney Area Health Service 2000). Interpreter availability was greater for the Tetum language than it had been for Albanian (South Western Sydney Area Health Service 2000).

The East Timorese retained their health records from Darwin. Information on follow-up needs and medication was supplied to receiving havens, as were health screening records and chest X-rays. However, despite lessons from the Kosovar experience regarding transfer of medical files, there were still some initial problems with this process.

Health issues

The medical needs of the East Timorese were generally greater than the Kosovars, necessitating the addition of a tent outside the clinic at one haven to increase the waiting area for patients (Roper 1999). Their situation was different in that Australia was their country of first asylum, and their evacuation occurred soon after exposure to highly traumatic events. The baseline standard of health and health care prior to the conflict was also lower than in Kosovo. Many East Timorese appeared frail, exhausted and/or malnourished on arrival. Cough and bronchitis were prominent, as were headache, chicken pox and other acute presentations. There was a considerably higher prevalence of tuberculosis (ten times the rate in the Kosovars), and several cases of malaria (Carrello et al. 2000; Roper 1999; South Western Sydney Area Health Service 2000). In addition to the acute illnesses, there was a high level of untreated chronic conditions and disability.

As with the Kosovars, immunisation was initially deferred until transfer to the safe havens. However, measles occurred among East Timorese in

Darwin and in two other havens. Vaccination of all evacuees aged between 9 months and 30 years was rapidly implemented as soon as cases appeared, as were various infection control measures. In Victoria visitors to the haven or excursions beyond the haven were not allowed until measles immunisations had been completed (Murphy undated). These events highlighted the need to implement measles immunisation early in an acute refugee emergency (Centers for Disease Control 1992; Médecins Sans Frontières 1997).

Demands on counselling services were greater among the East Timorese. This may have reflected the more recent nature of their psychological trauma, and the fact that those evacuated were directly threatened with violence prior to their sheltering in the UN compound, if not before. It may also have reflected their greater acceptance of emotional support through spiritual and other interventions.

The East Timorese began returning to their homeland on 28 October 1999. Most had left by the end of December that year.

Discussion and key lessons

Australia has been accepting migrants on a humanitarian basis since the end of World War II. In the early 1980s it was a country of first asylum for several thousand Vietnamese people arriving by boat, and continues to have a dedicated annual intake of refugees for resettlement. However, this was the first time that Australia had accepted evacuees airlifted directly from a crisis situation. Remarkably, this need arose twice in less than six months. The primary care approach adopted within the haven health services was overall a successful one. The support of specialised services and local hospitals was critical.

A multi-agency workshop to review the health aspects of Operation Safe Haven was convened by DHAC in December 1999. A number of key issues were identified:

1 Working in a multi-agency environment.

   The level of collaboration between agencies centrally and on the ground was high, but, at times, the different organisational cultures in such a wide variety of agencies led to differences in approach to some issues. Regular liaison meetings were vital for solving problems and developing agreed approaches.

2 The need for clear delineation of roles and responsibilities.

   Delays in establishing roles and responsibilities between the Commonwealth departments responsible for health and immigration caused some planning delays initially. Locally, roles and responsibilities of different agencies and individuals were not always clear, adding to the stress of workers on the ground. Delineation needs to occur early and be communicated clearly to all agencies and staff.

3   The need for better national coordination on health.

A lack of agreed communication protocols and of standardised surveillance and health status monitoring made it difficult for health staff to learn from the experience at other haven centres. A particular need identified was a method of uniquely identifying each evacuee to facilitate transfer of health information. The establishment of a specific committee to oversee health issues at a national level may have been beneficial. Health protocol updates could have been disseminated via a web site or email network, the latter having worked well at the local level and in the UK (Bowie 1999) in this situation. Regular teleconferences between haven centres would also have increased sharing of knowledge.

4   Short time frames.

The rapidity with which planning and implementation had to occur was difficult for all agencies and staff. This related to the initial implementation of the operation, the rapid turnaround times needed for medical screening and relocation interstate, and the organisation of repatriations. While the nature of refugee emergencies is such that short time frames are inevitable, early advice of central decisions, and rapid sharing of available information are vital for successful planning and implementation.

5   Staffing issues.

The uncertain duration of the project made permanent appointments difficult but the latter were more effective than sessional staff for maintaining continuity of care. The workloads of involved staff were significant, and care was needed to avoid burnout. Briefing of staff was useful to clarify role expectations, provide information about the health status of the population and to address cross-cultural issues. The provision of support and opportunities for debriefing for staff was important. Greater independence for nursing staff was a positive aspect, although adequate support was needed to avoid professional isolation. Volunteers from non-government organisations and from the haven communities were highly valued, despite some challenges in managing them.

6   Language barriers.

The importance of interpreters was one of the most constant issues raised. Frustration and inefficiencies were apparent due to competition between agencies for interpreter services and the limited number of medically trained interpreters. Active recruitment and adequate training of interpreters was seen as an important need. Demands on the interpreting staff were very high, support and debriefing for them being vital.

7 Logistic challenges.

Medical record collation and transfer was challenging throughout the entire Operation. Transportation of patients to hospital appointments worked better in some states than in others, the latter usually due to lack of clarity regarding which agency had responsibility. Food service provision required attention at several haven centres to ensure that adequate and culturally appropriate food was served, that food hygiene issues were addressed, and that the needs of small children were catered for.

8 Ethical challenges.

The restrictions placed on levels of health care funded by the Commonwealth reflected the temporary nature of the evacuees' stay. Health staff, however, found it difficult to refuse services to patients and many adopted the role of patient advocate, including assistance with identifying alternative sources of funding. The advocacy role and subsequent trusting relationship between staff and haven residents created ethical dilemmas during the repatriation phase, when medical staff were required to certify evacuees as being fit for return, despite the latter being fearful or having unmet medical needs.

Most health staff found the experience of working in such a setting highly valuable. Despite a number of challenges and frustrations, satisfaction with the work was strong, with a sense of having made a difference in assisting acutely traumatised people. Positive feedback from the haven residents added to the sense of accomplishment, and many staff expressed a willingness to be involved if such an event ever recurred.

Operation Safe Haven resulted from direct requests for assistance to the Australian Government from the United Nations in response to specific situations. While these situations are rare, the possibility of a recurrence can never be discounted. This overview of issues arising from health service provision during the 1999 operation can help inform planning for any such intervention in the future.

Acknowledgments

The information in this chapter was greatly enhanced by access to a large number of unpublished internal reports from a variety of different agencies. Their willingness to share such reports is greatly appreciated. Those contributing included:

- Commonwealth Department of Health and Ageing
- Department of Immigration and Multicultural and Indigenous Affairs
- Department of Human Services, Victoria
- Department of Human Services, South Australia
- Department of Health and Human Services, Tasmania
- Health Services Australia
- Hunter Area Health Service, NSW
- South Western Sydney Area Health Service, NSW
- Trauma Counselling Support Service, Tasmania
- Victorian Foundation for Survivors of Torture

Further thanks to Mr Aaron Silver and Ms Penny Roper for their assistance with gathering this information.

Recommended reading

Médecins Sans Frontières (1997) *Refugee Health: An approach to emergency situations*, Macmillan, London.

References

Ali, F., Gaukroger, M. & Swallow, M. (1999) Tasmanian Haven Centre Health Services—Summary Report. Debrief Workshop, Canberra, December 1999, Department of Health and Human Services, Tasmania, Hobart.

Bayman, R., Burton, G., D'Cruz, D. (2000) Operation Safe Haven—disaster recovery management with the Kosovar refugees: at Leeuwin Barracks, Western Australia, *Australian Journal of Emergency Management*, 15(1): 40–2.

Bennett, C., Mein, J., Beers, M., Harvey, B., Vemulpad, S., Chant, K. & Dalton, C. (2000) Operation Safe Haven: an evaluation of health surveillance and monitoring in an acute setting, *Communicable Diseases Intelligence*, 24(2): 21–6.

Bowie, C. (1999) The experience of serving the health needs of the refugees from Kosovo. A de-briefing report on the NHS response to the Kosovo Refugee Programme (unpublished), Department of Health, UK.

Carrello, C., Carr, B., Coleman, J. & Kolomyjec, C. (2000) Operation Safe Haven: the Leeuwin Experience, *Medical Journal of Australia*, 172: 502–5.

CDHAC (1999) Operation Safe Haven—Review of health aspects, Commonwealth Department of Health and Aged Care perspective, Commonwealth Department of Health and Aged Care, Canberra.

Centers for Disease Control (1992) Famine-affected, refugee and displaced populations: recommendations for public health issues, *MMWR Recommendations & Reports*, 41(RR-13): 1–76.

Centers for Disease Control and Prevention (1999) Health status of and Intervention for US bound Kosovar Refugees—Fort Dix, New Jersey, May–July 1999, *MMWR*, 48(33): 729–32.

Coombe, J. (2000) The Kosovar Experience in the Department of Human Services, SA, *Australian Journal of Emergency Management*, 15(1): 36–9.

Department of Human Services South Australia (1999) Operation Safe Haven—Adelaide Haven Centre: The Health Response, South Australian Department of Human Services, Adelaide.

DIMIA (1999a) Summary Report: Multiagency debriefing—Initial Reception Phase—Operation Safe Haven, August 1999 (draft unpublished), Department of Immigration and Multicultural and Indigenous Affairs (NSW), Sydney.

DIMIA (1999b) Workshop to review the health aspects of Operation Safe Haven (for Kosovar and East Timor evacuees), background papers, Department of Immigration and Multicultural and Indigenous Affairs, Canberra.

Health Services Australia (1999a) Flight Six to Sydney, In (ed), *Pulse—Your guide to health in the workplace. Special Kosovar Edition—1999*, Health Services Australia, Canberra.

Health Services Australia (1999b), personal communication.

McComb J. and Duquemin, A. (2001) Health in the East Timorese Tent City—the Territory Health Services response to the East Timorese evacuation, September 1999 Darwin, Territory Health Services, Darwin.

Médecins Sans Frontières (1997) *Refugee Health: An approach to emergency situations,* Macmillan, London.

Merriman, K. (1999), *Singleton Safe Haven Centre: Brief report of services provided by Hunter Area Health Service,* Hunter Area Health Service, Newcastle.

Murphy, C. (undated) Operation Safe Haven—the Victorian Perspective, Department of Human Services, Victoria, Melbourne.

National Health and Medical Research Council (NHMRC) (2000) *The Australian immunisation handbook*, NHMRC, Canberra.

National Health and Medical Research Council (NHMRC) (1995) *Protocol for health screening of boat people arriving in Australia*, NHMRC, Canberra.

National Public Health Partnership (1999) The Kosovars—The National Public Health Effort, *National Public Health Partnership News*, pp. 1–2.

PHLS (1999) The disease problems of Kosovan refugees in Albania, *CDR Weekly*, 9(18): 155.

Roper, P. (1999) Haven Health Services—Puckapunyal, Victoria, A Brief Overview, North Western Health Care Network, Melbourne.

Smith, M. (1999) Health implications for workers and volunteers of Operation Safe Haven, NSW Refugee Health Service, Sydney.

Smith, M., Comino, E., Williams, A., Harris, E. & Eagar, S. (2001) Kosovar & East Timorese evacuees in Sydney: a comparison of morbidity, In *Diversity in Health Conference*, Sydney 28–30 May, 2001.

South Western Sydney Area Health Service (2000) Operation Safe Haven—East Hills Centre: The Health Perspective, South Western Sydney Area Health Service, Sydney.

Stow, M. & Leary, R. (undated) The Work of the Foundation Teams in the Puckapunyal and Portsea Safe Havens, VFST, Melbourne.

Trauma Counselling Support Service (undated) Tasmanian Haven Centre—Review of Service, Trauma Counselling Support Service, Hobart.

10

A Thousand Yellow Envelopes: Providing Support to Temporary Protection Visa Refugees

Ainslie Hannan

On release from mandatory detention, the Temporary Protection Visa (TPV) refugee is given a public service yellow A1 envelope. The envelope contains thirty-eight pieces of crucial information (written, except for the occasional customer service number, in English); copies of completed, A, B and C Refugee Application Claim forms; map 43 of the central business district of Melbourne photocopied from the Melway and more forms such as an application for Medicare, just waiting to be completed. The envelope accompanies the TPV refugee everywhere, the forms and papers taken in and out of the envelope by the refugee, in the hope that their meaning will become apparent, or perhaps just out of some sense of nervousness that by somehow keeping these papers smooth and in order they will provide some sense of stability to feelings of temporariness.

Fundamental to the health and well-being of refugees is the hope and trust that after fleeing 'a well founded fear of persecution' (UNHCR 1951), they can finally rest and attain a different life in their country of asylum, Australia. In October 1999, the introduction of legislation creating TPVs resulted in a second class or under class of refugee. Under this legislation the refugees' rights are temporary; they have no access to settlement services, to return travel rights, or to family reunion. The policy and its conditions are constantly changing and underpinning the changing legislation is the need for containment and deterrence.

As the violation of trust is often at the core of the refugee experience, the impact of the TPV legislation on the health of this group of refugees cannot be overstated. The personal and community effects of this policy on asylum seekers is the subject of this chapter. As the coordinator of the Ecumenical Migration Centre in Melbourne, I started and continue to write a journal documenting conversations, incidents and voices from the shadows of public policy. Excerpts of this unpublished journal are used in this chapter to illustrate the health impacts of the Temporary Protection Visa Legislation not only the on health of the refugee but on all those who are in contact with it. (Because of issues of confidentiality the names and some of the particular detail is written as a collective account.)

Temporary protection: a policy of containment

On 13 October 1999 the Minister for Immigration and Multicultural and Indigenous Affairs Philip Ruddock, with bipartisan support, announced that unauthorised arrivals who are successful in their application for refugee status in Australia will no longer be granted permanent residence but instead be given three year Temporary Entry Visas (Visa Subclass 785). Asylum seekers who arrived lawfully will still be granted Permanent Residence Visas (Visa Subclass 866). Two classes of refugees have thus been created and both have very different entitlements. These are summarised in table 10.1.

A national strategy was established in 1996 in recognition that there were essential services that needed to be provided to refugees if their special needs were to be addressed. A key plank in the Australian Government's implementation of the TPV policy is to deny these refugees access to services and entitlements that form part of Australia's National Integrated Humanitarian Strategy on release from detention. Without access to the Settlement Support System, from July 2000, thousands of men, women, elderly, adolescent, and child refugees on TPVs, clutching their yellow envelopes were released from detention directly into the community.

The nature of the policy entails a heavy reliance on charity and community support for TPV refugees. The Brotherhood of St Laurence Ecumenical Migration Centre (EMC), assisted by a small grant from the Victorian State Government worked with welfare, local government and community/religious organisations to settle at times two busloads of refugees a week being released from detention. The EMC is a statewide, non-ethnospecific centre that works with recently arrived, emerging communities, as well as longer settled disadvantaged groups, to facilitate access and participation in Australian society. EMC delivers services and support structures for groups that are small in numbers, often dispersed and with complex needs as a result of the refugee experience. In the first six months the EMC opened 480 client files. They consisted of Afghan, Hazaras, Iranians, Kurds, and several 'stateless' people. EMC established

Table 10.1 Refugee visa entitlements

Service	Permanent Visa	Temporary Visa
Centrelink (Federal Government welfare organisation)	Immediate access to the full range of social security benefits	Access only to special benefits for which a range of eligibility criteria apply. Work test imposed.
Education	Some access to education like other permanent residents	Access to school education, subject to State policy. Effective preclusion from tertiary education due to imposition of full fees.
Settlement Support	Access to a full range of settlement support services offered provided by the Department of Immigration and Multicultural and Indigenous Affairs	No access to settlement services funded by Department of Immigration and Multicultural and Indigenous Affairs.
Family Reunion	Ability to bring members of immediate family (spouse and children) to Australia	No family reunion rights (including reunion with spouse and children).
Work Rights	Permission to work	Permission to work but ability to find employment influenced by temporary nature of their visa.
Language Training	Access to 510 hours of English language training	No access to English language classes funded by Department of Immigration and Multicultural and Indigenous Affairs.
Medical Benefits	Automatic eligibility for Medicare	Eligibility for Medicare subject to lodgment.
Travel	Ability to leave the country and return without jeopardising their visa	No return travel.

Refugee Council of Australia/Refugee Legal Service/ Ecumenical Migration Centre 2002

and coordinated that statewide housing and material aid database at times providing housing for seventy refugees a week. The immediate need was to establish a crisis intervention system.

Over time and with strong partnerships including those from the Justice for Asylum Seeker Alliance, a more coordinated and less reactive response has been developed in Victoria. Despite this the uncertainty that the TPV has been designed to bring and as more refugees continue to be released from detention into the care of new arrival communities, the informal service system with its Federal Government placed restrictions becomes exhausted and resources become depleted. New challenges continue to appear, which makes the health of these refugees, the communities that support them and the health of the whole Australian society fragile and sometimes critical. The health impacts of the temporary protection legislation stretches beyond those immediately involved. It diminishes all Australians, as the mark of any civilised society is how it treats its most vulnerable.

It is important to note that health and well-being will be affected by the potential material deprivation and restricted access to public goods imposed by the TPV policy. In addition however, any discussion of the health impacts of the legislation on refugees needs to address the individual experience of the refugee and the impact of the policy on their particular life situation. The magnitude of the impact of the TPV legislation on the health of refugees is in the translation of the policy to the individual and family experience. The following experience illustrates the effect of the lack of travel rights and family reunion.

Do you have the list? I ask the Iraqi community leader as he sits still next to me. We have sat together many times over the past two years. My question makes me feel intrusive. The Brotherhood of St Laurence is administering a small fund established by a private donor who has collected money as a gesture of support to surviving family members whose relatives drowned off the coast of Java in October 2001. Abdul slides a piece of paper that looks like it has been torn from a note pad and has been carried with him in his wallet for the last week. Nine family names written in blue ink, in Arabic from right to left with numbers alongside them. The numbers relate to how many people from each family had drowned. Many had lost their wife and all of their children. Others had lost up to sixteen immediate and all of their extended family. 'Why so many Iraqis?' I ask Abdul. As his fingertip outlines the names he looks down, grief stricken, he utters, 'Iraqis have large families and this was a cheap boat'. They were desperate; there was no choice. Men from Preston who had already been granted Temporary Protection Visas went back to Indonesia to help their terrified wives and children make the trip across the sea. The constantly changing Temporary Protection Visa legislation with no family reunion and not even an opportunity of return travel rights to ensure the safety of their families provides few choices for those on Temporary Protection Visas.

(Hannan, journal notes, March 2002)

The reactivity of the policy and frequent changes in the legislation meant that the refugee does not have the opportunity to feel settled. Centrelink data reveals that out of the 1020 TPV refugees on special benefits in Melbourne and Sydney, there are fifty people moving between Melbourne and Sydney at any given time. The need for employment is so great that there is significant movement to and across rural Victoria. Twenty-seven per cent of all TPV refugees live in country Victoria. As this figure does not include dependent children or those in employment the figure is likely to be significantly higher.

The impact of the fluidity of the legislation is constant; the reaches of the legislation are never static as its restrictions expand so as to contain new situations as they arise. Hope can't always be diminished. It needs to have some relief so that it can rebuild trust as illustrated below.

> Marsoud changes his name to Mark and lives with an Australian family. Hope pushes his depression back. He does not talk about his family left behind in hiding in Iraq waiting for him. He decided not to live in transitional housing with the other men who had been with him for his thirteen months in detention. He starts to understand the implications for him of being on a TPV; he has purchased an international phone card in the hope of some contact with his wife overseas. His body is starting to visibly loose its hold on depression as he counts down the thirty months on his visa until he can apply for permanent residency, and then in time family reunion. He stands straight the resilience of hope that life can be different is building.
>
> (Hannan, journal notes, August 2001)

Then in September 2001, seven new laws were rushed through parliament again changing the conditions for Mark and all refugees on Temporary Protection Visas. The Migration Legislation Amendment Act 2001, in addition to giving the Australian Government further powers to prevent asylum seekers from landing in Australia; further restricted asylum seekers' right of appeal; removed parts of Australia from the Australian immigration zone and also defined a new Australian visa regime. This regime with its hierarchy of rights is intended to deter further movement from, or bypassing of, other 'safe' countries. Those who make their claims in refugee camps and are approved by the Office of the United Nations High Commissioner for Refugees (UNCHR) are given permanent resident status. Those who are settled in Australia from transit countries (such as Indonesia, a country that is arguably inhospitable to many asylum seekers) may be granted a Temporary Protection Visa, but will not be eligible for the grant of a permanent visa for four-and-a-half years. Those who reach Australia, apart from directly fleeing persecution within their country of origin, will only be eligible for successive temporary visas.

> Mark comprehends the changes to the legislation. Like a ghost haunted by his shadow of diminished hope wearing fragility in his eyes Mark utters, 'I don't

want to be called a refugee any more. Why can't I just be a friend needing a place to go? I don't know why Australians don't realise. We can't go back. When we climbed on to that boat, taking the hand of the smuggler, we formed a suicide pact. Self hatred has filled us from the time we knew that the Australian or any other navy might let us drown in the sea. This will never leave us; we wake up every morning knowing that you don't want us. But we have no choice but to risk our lives and throw ourselves at your mercy'.

(Hannan, journal notes, October 2001)

Before the revised regulations (some six months after the release of the first refugees from detention), refugees on TPVs were not eligible for a Medicare card until they had submitted their application for permanent protection. If the refugee did not know where to seek the limited volunteer lawyer support to complete their application they did it themselves. Sometimes this application was completed in the refugee's first language of Arabic or Dari and at times the application was lodged with the Department of Immigration and Multicultural and Indigenous Affairs with whole sections blank. In the main this was done with the refugees' knowledge that their application was incomplete and that this had potentially serious implications for their application for permanent residency. However, there was often some urgency for the process to be completed because many health issues were not brought to the attention of authorities while in detention because of a lack of trust. On release many of these conditions require immediate attention, necessitating an expedition of the process required to make this possible.

Currently full Medicare eligibility is available upon application to all refugees on a TPV. However, delays of six weeks or more have been experienced with processing of applications and some cards have been issued for an interim period only, needing reissuing. In the initial stages staff at suburban Medicare offices in Melbourne had received no training regarding the entitlements of refugees on temporary protection and in the main they did not access interpreters to clarify enquiries. The result was that some went away without Medicare cards. In a few cases assistance was sought from a hospital for what had become a health emergency. Fees were then charged based on consultations of international patients, a rate that was prohibitive to TPV refugees.

The effects of these difficulties are evident at multiple levels as Mohammed describes.

Mohammed, having been released from the Curtin Detention Centre five days earlier was ill; he was distraught with worry. He could not move his arms. They were full with tremendous pain. As yet he had no Medicare card. Smith

Street Collingwood, a July winter's day, well after 7pm. Mohammed and I had been with each other for the previous five hours, waiting for a free emergency medical appointment that had been provided by a sympathetic Community Health Centre. Now we were explaining to the pharmacist how it was that Mohammed was receiving a Special Benefit payment from Centrelink but still had no pharmaceutical concession card. We walk together from the chemist to the car, night has fallen, and Mohammed almost reminiscent in a soft voice speaks of his wife and three children hiding, waiting for him on the Pakistani border. You know you remind me of my wife she is always organising me. I smile and respond to his earlier question about where to purchase thongs, as he can't stand the heat of his feet in his laced up boots. I explain that you can buy them in the $2 shop and I then go on to explain cheap alternative shopping in Melbourne. I suggest that seeing that it is just next door that we may as well just go and get a pair. Mohammed stops and looks at me and asserts, no please just take me home. I am surprised by this almost hostile response I ask whether he is ok? Mohammed looks me dead in the eyes, now even more withdrawn he states; I was tortured in Afghanistan. I nearly drowned at the hands of the smugglers. I was then placed in your detention camps for almost fourteen months where my hair fell out. Others from Woomera developed white spots on their skin but still they could not get fresh water or medical care. I was released from the Curtin Detention Centre with only two hours notice and no opportunity to say goodbye. I have been on a bus for sixty hours arriving here in Melbourne with no information on what is likely to happen next. I have now been told today by a doctor that the pain in my arms is not physical and perhaps if I take sedatives in time and with rest the pain will leave me? How can I ever be completely open with you? I need to survive. I can not afford to or to let you unravel my heart

(Hannan, car conversation with Mohammed, journal notes, August 2001)

In a fifteen-month period and for many, after more than eight months in detention, 3949 refugees were released into the community in 2001. The ongoing damage to the health of these refugees on TPVs needs to be understood in the context of their whole refugee experience. Many, before arriving in Australia have been tortured and remain traumatised; unlike other refugees arriving in Australia they are placed in mandatory detention for unlimited and often extended periods of time.

Many refugees in Woomera were mentally unwell and had nightmares. The harsh conditions and the uncertainty about the duration of their stay in detention, long waiting periods to hear about their cases made them anxious that they would be deported. People were scared and you need to understand the Taliban had already made us scared. We arrived with fear. In the night at Woomera we would hear men, many of whom were boys, wake with fright from their nightmares. We would hear their sobs in the stillness of the night. The woman sitting slightly behind her husband looks at me as she says: The cries of the men would wake our children. Our children cried the whole time we were in detention. They would not play with the toys.

(Hannan, journal notes, 2001)

The long-term health effects of detaining refugees and then only giving them temporary protection is yet to be determined. Sultan and O'Sullivan (2001) report in their analysis of Australian detention centres, that the psychological reaction patterns of detainees who wait for extended periods of time while their claims for asylum are assessed are characterised by stages of increasing depression, punctuated by periods of protest, as feelings of injustice overwhelm them.

Sitting opposite, Fatima leans towards me. After nine months in detention she now lives across the road in transitional high rise accommodation. She has not as yet been granted public housing. She cares for twelve-year-old second son Ali. Because of insufficient funds to pay the smugglers Ali's older brother has been left in Iraq to care for his four remaining siblings. Together Ali and his mother made the hazardous journey to flee Iraq; the journey started eighteen months ago. Fatima is worried, she looks at me with her dark still eyes as she explains, Ali won't settle at the language school. There are days when he refuses to go. I thought going to school again would make him happy. Ali went to school for a while in a portable at Woomera. Then one day at Woomera, as I was looking out of the paneless window, I saw my son standing on the yellow dust in the middle of the compound looking to the sky. He was begging to the moving clouds, crying, as if searching for freedom. School without warning had been cancelled for the day. This had been enough to destabilise him. I stood there frozen. I had nothing to offer him. I could not go to him. Each of his tears burnt my heart. I just watched him, somehow instinctively knowing that hunt for freedom. Ali never went back to school at Woomera.

(Hannan, interview with Fatima at the EMC, journal notes, February 2002)

Hope and refugees

Hope is central to the refugee recovery process. Hope is the ability in times of absolute human trial not to give up on life, to hold on to the belief in your own and others' ability to be compassionate. Hope is not wishful thinking; hope is based on a framework of justice, a memory or an experience that somehow life can be different. This is not to say that hope is not fragile and at times needs to be fuelled by the imagination. For the refugee the breadth and the size of the imagination that can be transported and safely constructed by hope become essential equipment for their health and well-being. This imagination may contain the seeds for trust to start to flourish, or it may include souvenirs that will encourage memories of resilience, fuel for the imagination of hope that they and their families will be able to once again live in individual freedom. There is little hope offered by the TPV policy that exacerbates the fragility of the refugees' hope.

Another restriction on rights that affected health and well-being included employment. Refugees reported that because of their TPV they were often denied employment as employers did not understand the visa and did not want to employ someone temporarily. Or as in Mohammed's case an unscrupulous employer employed him without award conditions or Workcover entitlements and put him on a 16-hour shift, six days a week. Desperate for money and not knowing his entitlements Mohammed worked in that factory—pulling skins across barrels until his finger nails bled and his hands were paralysed with pain (Hannan, journal notes, September 2001).

A thousand yellow envelopes—from crisis to intervention

Do you know who we are? Sunday night, July 2000—he sat opposite me in the Brotherhood of St Laurence car. His fellow countrymen sat silently in the back seat pointing to the streetlights. We drove from the Preston Mosque where they had slept the previous night with forty-two others on the floor. Two days earlier they had been released from the Woomera Detention Centre with just two hours notice. Whilst on the bus they had been advised that the State Department of Immigration and Multicultural Affairs in Melbourne, would book one night's accommodation for them in a backpackers inn. They would receive an unstipulated amount of money when they got off the bus, this was to last until they received their first Centrelink payment. Once in the backpackers inn in Bourke St Melbourne they became completely disorientated and were too frightened by the behaviour of the other backpacker residents to leave their rooms. Community groups and welfare agencies like the Brotherhood of St Laurence and the Islamic Council of Victoria stepped in to support the recently arrived Afghan and Iraqi communities who had been made responsible for the settlement of all refugees from their community's being released from detention. As we drove to an Anglicare Emergency family accommodation house, that had just been painted and so fortunately was vacant, his eyes underneath his backward baseball cap intensely scrutinised me to see whether a plank of trust could be formed. His intense eyes, the rigidity of his unwell looking body signalled his desperate need to explain his refugee case, to be believed. Do you know who we are? He persisted. We are the Hazara. Since 1649 Afghanistan and the Hazara people have a whole series of different histories of persecution. Our latest history is about the Taliban. The Taliban systematically and ruthlessly kills the Hazara. We are the Hazara people we have few choices. The Hazaras are like the thorns on the roses that have to be picked off so that the Taliban can hold the roses. Despite my fifteen-year experience of working with refugees until now I had never heard of the Hazara.

(Hannan, car conversation with Ali, journal notes, July 2001)

The response to the release of detainees included twice weekly pre-arrival work with community leaders, and agencies to confirm with the Department of Immigration and Multicultural and Indigenous Affairs the numbers of arrivals to be released into Victoria. Ethnicity, family com position, the numbers of minors all needed to be ascertained so that the necessary response services could be put into place. This crisis intervention system included everything from finding and coordinating temporary accommodation to seemingly small but crucial tasks of photocopying the relevant map from the Melway so that the location of the accommodation could be explained to each refugee.

Once the pre-arrival work was completed, the on-arrival work was then coordinated. This included the opening of case files for each refugee and where necessary placing different coloured dots on case files signalling the need for additional services. For example a red dot signalled significant health issues, a green dot that the refugee was an unattached minor. The opening of case files ensured that there was a mechanism that could be used to record the allocation of temporary accommodation so as to reunite refugees who were later released from detention. Each case file contained a checklist of all the documents each refugee should have in their yellow envelope as some refugees had been released from detention without all of their crucial documents. The checklist provided a way to document necessary follow-up work. The case files were also used to hold key documents including a formal record of receipt and handover of mailed or received documents. The file was a place to hold important mail as it was common for the refugees to move from one house to another reuniting with friends or reflecting an inability to settle.

Central to the coordination of the settlement of the Temporary Protection Visa refugees was the finding, training, and coordination of bilingual groups of volunteers and the supervision of social work students. The volunteers and students would accompany EMC staff to the reception centres to welcome the busloads of refugees who had often been travelling all night from Australia's remote detention centres. Each volunteer or student would accompany each family or group of refugees to their emergency accommodation. As part of this role they ensured that the family or household of single men understood things like how to switch on the power; the location of halal shops; how to get assistance in an emergency and how to find their way back to the EMC in three days time for an information session. The compassion and care shown by the volunteers and students gave a very strong message of welcome to the refugees who reported that except for their initial naval rescue they had felt unwelcome. The volunteers' and students' attention to detail had a very important positive impact on the health of the refugees. As it was necessary to have a relevant language, volunteers often needed to be drawn from newly arrived, under-resourced communities. Despite the enormous commitment, over time these communities became over stretched and exhausted.

The preliminary supervised assessment conducted by the student and bilingual volunteers at the reception centres was followed up at the twice weekly information sessions held at the Ecumenical Migration Centre. In addition to assessing whether the refugees had issues that required an immediate emergency response, the sessions provided vital settlement information. The information included everything from how to open a bank account and how the health/welfare and tax system operates in Australia, to their legal and visa obligations and group discussions where their immediate health and welfare needs were assessed. As part of the information session each refugee was referred to a more detailed health session facilitated by the Victorian Foundation for the Survivors of Torture.

Tuesday afternoon at the Ecumenical Migration Centre the tea is being made, whilst what feels like hundreds of men, women and children, holding on to their yellow envelops, desperately engage with each other in Dari or in Arabic. As a strategy to cope with the sheer volume of need, after the general information session, people are asked to form language groups of no more than ten. Groups are formed quickly as people are eager to get assistance. I recognise some of the faces from the previous week. Many return to each information session to either hear the information again or in the hope of greeting a friend who has been recently released from detention. I sit with a social work student and an interpreter surveying the group in front of me in the hope of recognising an issue before it is too late. I apologise for the need to talk with people in a small group. I explain that if there is a need, it is also possible for people to speak to me individually. I explain the role of the welfare state in Australia, the role of the social worker and of confidentiality. As I explain once again that the EMC is not the Government I feel, except for the enormity of the tragedy, that I am somehow part of a John Cleese film. As my eyes connect with the eyes of the ten men, women and children sitting in front of me I state once again that the Ecumenical Migration Centre as an organisation and that I as individual deeply regret Australia's detention and temporary protection policy. Follow-up sheets are used to document issues from individuals in the group. By the end of the group session each sheet reads like a litany of abuse from lost family members, to ongoing nightmares provoked by the fear of the unknown, to desperate requests for assistance to enroll their children into school. Towards the end of the group session I ask whether anyone has any immediate health issues that need attention prior to their Medicare cards being processed. Ardil has been sitting quietly; he now leans forward, putting his hands on the table as he pushes his shirtsleeves up one at a time. He looks me dead in the eyes. The other group members sit back knowing what he will reveal. Ardil's arms from the elbow down had been broken and have reset themselves backwards. As my tear-filled eyes connect with his tearful eyes he utters, Please can you help me? I cannot bear the pain.

(Hannan, group work discussion, journal notes, August 2001)

Every wall of the Ecumenical Migration Centre was strewn with lists of emergency accommodation options. On each list, names of the Temporary Protection Visa refugees who had been allocated to the property were listed. There were rooms that had been given in case of an emergency, but only for one night; private houses given by people who were about to holiday overseas from ordinary Australians who had telephoned to offer support, expressing their shame to be Australians, generously offering their houses and emergency assistance as a way to send a contrasting message of compassion to the refugee families released from detention. There were lists of names on doors in Arabic and Dari signalling that mail had arrived. Kitchens and offices were full with overwhelmed, exhausted volunteers and community leaders. As they were often new arrival refugees themselves they were desperate to get advice and information so that they could provide meaningful assistance. The strain and responsibility of settling so many men, women and children with such complex needs was affecting their own health and well-being. Until a system was established there was an almost constant sense of being drowned by the demands of what were desperate fearful people on temporary protection. The limitations of such a reactive response was that with every health crisis presented there was an increasing feeling of staggering from one crisis to another. At times it felt like the health needs were so enormous that they were at best under-managed or unmanaged.

In order to prevent the crisis intervention framework and to avoid the creation of new crises, a more coordinated response was developed by July 2001. Experience, statewide and regional partnerships and the sheer reduction in numbers of refugees being released from detention has meant that intelligent problem solving has informed a more coordinated community response. The Victorian State Government allocated small grants to the regions and rural Victoria. This sent a very powerful message of support. Regional responses were established. The Ecumenical Migration Centre continues its support to families on TPVs, community leaders, and to the regions. The EMC has an ongoing role in developing systems and convening statewide meetings to provide support, to document ongoing issues and to ensure the maximum cooperation of critical services like material aid. Statewide meetings of community leaders and service providers document the emerging health needs of refugees on TPVs and of those who support them. Although there is now a greater coordinated intervention response there remains an ongoing need for an immediate crisis response to still be possible.

Recommended reading

International Catholic Migration Commission (2001) Futures of refugees and refugee resettlement, *International Journal of Refugee Law*, 13(4): 569–83.
Jones, D. & Gill, P. (1998) Refugees and primary care: tackling the inequalities, *British Medical Journal*, 317: 1444–6.
UNHCR and Victorian Foundation for Survivors of Torture (VFST, 2002) *Refugee resettlement: an international handbook to guide reception and integration*, UNHCR, Geneva.

References

Hannan, A. (2001) Voices from the shadow of public policy, *Migration Action*, XXIII (1).
Sultan, A. & O'Sullivan, K. (2001) Psychological disturbances in asylum seekers held in long term detention: a participant—observer account, *Medical Journal of Australia*, 175: 593–6.
UNHCR (1951) Convention relating to the status of refugees, UNHCR, Geneva.

11

The Health of Young Asylum Seekers and Refugees in the United Kingdom: Reflection from Research

Astier M. Almedom and Rachael Gosling

Introduction

The terms 'asylum seeker' and 'refugee' lend themselves to a wide range of interpretations depending on the political, social, legal and ethical/moral contexts in which they are used. In their own words, refugees are people who 'have been forced to leave home', 'with nowhere to go', 'cannot go home', or 'have no home' (Penz 2000; Petty & Jareg 1998; Summerfield 1997). In the United Kingdom (UK), the difference between an asylum seeker and a refugee is one of status: the former is a person who has applied for refugee status and is waiting for the Home Office (HO) to decide, while the latter is a person who has been granted refugee status in accordance with Article 1 of the Geneva Convention and Protocol (UNHCR 1951, 1967). Asylum applications lodged in the UK constitute 16.5 per cent of the total number lodged in Europe, North America, Australia and New Zealand from 1999 to 2001 (UNHCR 2002).

This chapter presents an example of health service research and development aimed at improving the health and well-being of young refugees in the South London boroughs of Lambeth, Southwark, and Lewisham. The role of practice-led, action orientated research in determining what the needs are, what is already being done to meet existing needs, and what can be done to maximise the strengths and address weaknesses of existing systems is discussed. The journey of asylum seeking in the UK is outlined with respect to its impact on the health of children and young people. Existing linkages and disparities between national and international humanitarian policy and public health are explored, and it is argued that

1993: Asylum and Immigration Appeals Act
- the 1951 UN Refugee Convention and 1967 Protocol enshrined in UK law
- rejected asylum seekers given the right of appeal within strict time limits
- all asylum seekers, including children required to be fingerprinted
- asylum seekers entitled to welfare benefits (though income support paid at 90%)

1996: Asylum and Immigration Act
- asylum seekers applying at port of entry entitled to receive welfare benefits
- asylum seekers applying after arrival, 'in-country' applicants, not entitled to receive welfare benefits. As a result of this legislation, local social service departments were obliged to provide 'food and shelter' to 'destitute' in-country applicants under the National Assistance Act, 1948
- introduction of 'White List' of countries
- fast-track system introduced for asylum seekers from 'white list' countries and those with 'manifestly unfounded' applications
- restrictions on employment of asylum seekers and introduction of fines for employers found to be employing people without permission to work. Asylum seekers could apply for permission to work after residence in the UK for six months

1999: Asylum Act
- removal of all rights to welfare benefits from asylum seekers and introduction of voucher system. Vouchers could be exchanged for food and basic goods in certain supermarkets and were valued at 70% of income support
- National Asylum Support Service (NASS) created within the Home Office to provide financial support to all asylum seekers, except unaccompanied children
- asylum seekers 'dispersed' on a no-choice basis from London and the south-east to other parts of the UK, such as Glasgow, Leeds, and Liverpool
- aimed to reduce the time taken to process applications to six months
- introduction of an 'integration strategy' for people with refugee status and Exceptional Leave to Remain

2002: Asylum and Immigration Bill—Proposals
- voucher system replaced by a cash system, administered by NASS (this came into force in April 2002)
- introduction of identity cards for asylum seekers (already being phased in)
- agreement of a bilateral resettlement program with United Nations High Commissioner for Refugees (UNHCR)
- introduction of a national network of 'induction centres', situated near ports of entry, each providing full board accommodation for 200 to 400 asylum seekers, during their first seven days in the UK
- open four 'accommodation centres', each providing full board accommodation to 750 asylum seekers (including children), while their claims for asylum are processed. The success of the accommodation centres to be evaluated. Children of asylum seekers will not be allowed to attend local schools
- introduction of 'removal centres', where asylum seekers whose applications have been rejected are detained, prior to their deportation
- dispersal away from London and the south-east to continue for those not in accommodation centres
- asylum seekers will not be allowed to work until a decision on their application has been made (effective 23 July 2002)

Figure 11.1 Chronology of UK legislation pertaining to asylum seekers

UK government reforms in public health policy and practice are well intended and operationally complex; while asylum/immigration policy and practice are problematic on humanitarian grounds. This has a negative impact on the health and well-being of asylum seekers and refugees, particularly children and young people.

Asylum and immigration policy and practice in the UK

Prior to 1993, legislation that referred specifically to asylum seekers did not exist in the UK. Up to that time, large-scale arrivals had included 17,000 Hungarians in 1956; 37,000 Ugandans in 1972; 24,000 Cypriots in 1974; and 27,500 Somalis in 1988 (Refugee Council 1999). The first legislation concerning asylum seekers was passed in 1993. Since then, three major Acts of Parliament have been passed, with the fourth receiving Royal Assent on 7 November 7 2002—the Nationality, Immigration and Asylum Act 2002. The main features of each Act are summarised in figure 11. 1.

A review of recent statistics published by the United Nations High Commissioner for Refugees (UNHCR), the Refugee Council, and the HO reveals that between 1999 and 2001, the UK ranked twelfth out of twenty-five European countries in asylum applications lodged per 1000 inhabitants (UNHCR 2002). In 2001, 28,040 of the 71,700 asylum applicants were from Iraq, Afghanistan, Somalia, and Sri Lanka. The majority were allowed temporary admission, while others were detained and/or deported. On 30 March 2002, 1370 asylum seekers were in detention. A third of asylum applicants whose cases were decided received a positive decision in 2001 (this figure does not include positive decisions granted at appeal level, estimated by the Refugee Council to be a further 20 per cent of cases); and 9185 asylum seekers whose claims for asylum were rejected were deported or had returned voluntarily in 2001. Figure 11.2 illustrates the asylum seeker's journey in the UK.

Exceptional Leave to Remain (ELR) is granted to people who do not strictly meet the criteria of a refugee but are allowed to remain in the UK for humanitarian reasons. If ELR is granted, restrictions are placed on family reunion, travel abroad and access to higher education. ELR is granted for four years after which the applicant can request 'Indefinite Leave to Remain'. Once refugee status is granted, the option is open to apply for British citizenship.

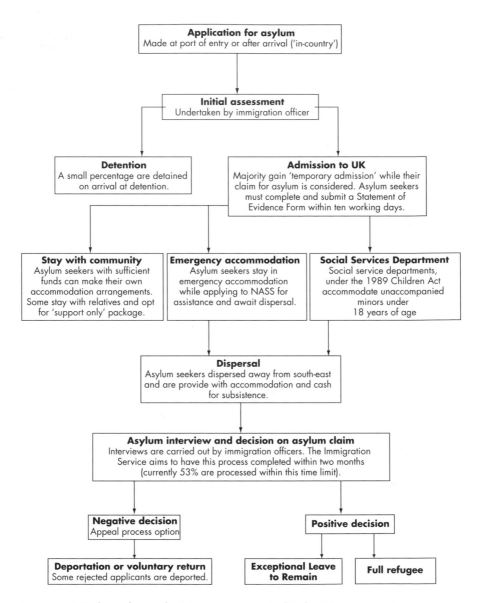

Figure 11.2 The asylum seeker's journey upon arrival in the UK

Enhancing public health policy and practice: the Health Action Zones

When New Labour took office in 1997, various initiatives to tackle poverty, social exclusion, and ill health were introduced. The Department of Health (DOH) called for detailed health improvement plans from each Health Authority (HA) and announced the Health Action Zone (HAZ) initiative, inviting Health Authorities, with demonstrable multi-agency partnerships in place to bid (Dean 1998; Department of Health 1997). The HAZ is a seven-year initiative of geographically defined target-orientated programs governed by a partnership board that includes local statutory and non-statutory agencies in the health, social, education, and humanitarian sectors.

The focus of the HAZ for Lambeth, Southwark, and Lewisham (LSL) was on children and young people (to age 25). It employed a holistic approach in which families and communities were included in the multi-sectoral programs of work on a variety of local priority areas such as reduction of teenage pregnancy, improved parenting, improved access to services and employment opportunities for disabled children and young people, and social inclusion of black and minority ethnic as well as other marginalised groups. Multi-agency working groups oversee and support HAZ work programs and priority areas. A preliminary report of the external evaluation describes the processes whereby HAZ activities are contributing to 'Whole Systems Change' (Hewitt et al. 2001).

In addition, a HAZ Innovation Fund (announced by the DOH in 1999, to accelerate the process of reform begun by the HAZ) was awarded to Community Health South London, a key HAZ stakeholder, for its 'Young Refugee Project'. The research presented in this chapter was conducted in order to assess how best to improve the health of young refugees by facilitating their access to services, possibly by employing 'link workers'.

Research aims and objectives

The aim was to gather first-hand data on the needs of young refugees in LSL in order to inform the HAZ National Innovation Fund's 'Young Refugee Project'. The general objectives were:

- to initiate multi-agency working as a first step to establishing a steering group representing the local health trusts, education departments, social services and voluntary agencies through the research process itself
- to ensure that young refugees were consulted appropriately so that the project could take into account their expressed needs

The specific objectives were:

- to produce a report which will contain recommendations on a strategy to improve the health of young refugees in LSL and to facilitate their access to local services
- to engage key stakeholders and receive their input in the development of phase two of the project

For the purposes of this research, refugee children and young people were defined as 0 to 19 year olds living in the UK as refugees, asylum seekers, or with 'Exceptional Leave to Remain'. The research questions were:

- How many refugee children and young people are living in the district?
- What concerns do young refugees have about their health?
- What is their experience of accessing services?
- Would young refugees benefit from the input of link workers?
- How do local agencies respond to the needs of young refugees?
- To what extent do local agencies cooperate in responding to the needs of the young refugees?
- What are the gaps in service provision?
- Why do these gaps exist?

Participants and methods

Research was carried out over a total period of six months (January to June 2000). Data collection was primarily through individual interviews and focus group discussions with some mailed out questionnaires.

Individual interviews and discussions were conducted with a total of 26 key informants including local authority officers (social exclusion department officers, equality officers, asylum seeker team workers, education welfare officers and school improvement advisers), refugee health team members, community paediatricians, health visitors, and employees of voluntary organisations. Interviews were conducted informally at various times during the course of the research in order to find out who was doing what, and to identify possible roles for the link workers.

A total of thirty-three young refugees between the ages of 12 and 16 from each of the three boroughs participated in three focus group discussions. The focus group discussions were held in secondary schools. The schools' English language teachers selected pupils who could participate on the basis of their ability to express themselves in English (Somali, Albanian, and Arabic interpreters were present in one group, Group 2). The profile of the focus group discussion participants is outlined in table 11.1.

Table 11.1 Profile of focus group discussion participants (young refugees)

	Focus group one	Focus group two	Focus group three
Group size	13	12	8
Age	12–16	12–16	12–16
Length of time in the UK	6 months–3 years	3 months–11 years	4 months–most of life
Sex	4 girls and 9 boys	2 girls and 10 boys	All girls
Country of origin	Kosovo, Croatia, Afghanistan, Ivory Coast, Sri Lanka, Iran, Morocco, Jamaica, Congo	Mostly Kosovo (75%), Somalia, Morocco	Ghana, Kosovo, Iraq, Uganda, Pakistan, Somalia

Chairs of Primary Care Groups (PCG), school nurse professional supervisors, health visitor professional supervisors, education department officials, refugee community leaders, voluntary organisation workers, and youth workers were interviewed over the telephone using questionnaires. A total of 45 people were interviewed in this way.

Written surveys were used to elicit information from 178 respondents including general practitioners, school nurses, health visitors, dentists and social workers. Observation of existing projects, such as the 'Barnardos drop-in' for families in temporary accommodation most of whom were refugees, and a newly established 'one stop shop' organised by social services for asylum seekers in Lambeth, were conducted. Data were collated from various group discussions that took place during project based workshops.

Research findings

Based on the Neighbourhood Statistics Dataset, 1991 census data, the total population of children under the age of 16 in Lambeth, Southwark and Lewisham in 1998 was projected to be approximately 165,200. It was estimated that there were at least 7000 refugee children from a range of nationalities living in LSL. It was difficult to obtain accurate figures because of the multiple changes in government policy, which over the years had created different groups of refugees financially supported under a variety of disparate systems (see figure 11.3). Most practitioners who participated in the research did not routinely collect data on asylum seekers or refugees, either because they were not required to do so, or they felt that this would jeopardise the development of a trusting relationship

- Agencies that monitor refugees are those responsible for financially supporting them: social services, housing departments, benefits agencies, National Asylum Support Service. The data they collect are not collated. Some refugees and asylum seekers are not financially supported by any agency, so they do not appear in statistics.
- A number of London councils accommodate asylum seekers in other boroughs within and beyond the London region and these figures are difficult to establish.
- Many service providers do not record the immigration status of their service users.
- There is no clear definition of when a refugee stops being a refugee; this is often a question of self-perception.
- A percentage of asylum seekers whose applications have been rejected 'go underground'.
- Some asylum seekers and refugees are reluctant to identify themselves to government and other public institutions for a variety of reasons.
- Home Office statistics of asylum seekers show 'principal applicants' and do not include dependants. This adds to the difficulty of estimating the number of children. (Special efforts were made to ensure that all children, including newborn babies were included in the 2000 Census that will be released in September 2002. This may not show those whose immigration status is unknown.)
- The Home Office does not release data about where people live.

Figure 11.3 Difficulties encountered in establishing numbers of refugees in the three boroughs of Lambeth, Southwark, and Lewisham

between themselves and the client. This was explained by two respondents (professionals) as follows

> We don't ask [immigration] status—we do not want to frighten people and our primary concern is education.
>
> A teacher

> You just back off and don't ask those questions
>
> A health professional

Many asylum seekers are not aware of their entitlement to free health care and to education for their children, so accessing these services can be accompanied by feelings of insecurity and fear. Community thoracic nurse interviewees reported that they had learnt from experience that asking people their immigration status can jeopardise their attendance at clinic for on-going treatment. This presents significant difficulties for planning and funding services.

The young refugees and the professionals who participated in this research identified a range of factors, some of which are specific to the refugee experience, as having an influence on their health and well-being, and their access to services. Many of the young refugees interviewed were living in poverty, in substandard, insecure, and overcrowded housing. Some talked about not having enough money to buy clothes or food. Others experienced the insecurity and disruption of frequent moves from one hostel to another. This aspect of refugee life was also discussed by professionals who were struggling to track refugees who would suddenly disappear from their service, without notification. Important information regarding an individual's health is lost as health professionals are not informed when or where refugees move. Health workers had also seen patients who walked long distances to clinics because they did not have money for public transport.

Concern was voiced by professionals about the mental health of young refugees and the lack of specialist services to respond appropriately. All the young refugees interviewed had experienced separation from family members and some were unaccompanied minors, living in foster care. A 13-year-old unaccompanied minor from Uganda explained that she was in poor health because 'I have so many worries and problems'.

A common feature among the young refugees who participated in the focus group discussions was loneliness and this was compounded by their experience at school, where they were bullied and in some cases, physically attacked by other children. Very few knew about local youth clubs or community groups. Some expressed concern about the health of their parents and had taken on an adult role within the family, due to their more rapid acquisition of English. A 12-year-old girl from Iraq explained:

> If you are the only person to speak English, it makes you feel like an adult, not a child. It's like if you leave, everyone else will fall down.

It was also found that professionals often use refugee children to interpret for their relatives to overcome the language barrier and to compensate for an inadequate interpreting service. Some young people revealed that they had taken time off school to accompany a parent or relative to a doctor's appointment.

The young refugees also articulated the factors that had a positive effect on their health. These included having a good doctor, being in a country with a 'good medical system', being able to eat good food, being able to learn English and having friends. However, despite these positives, many felt that their health had deteriorated since their arrival in the UK (Gosling 2000a).

Most of the young refugees interviewed had accessed primary health care services and were registered with their local general practitioner (GP), although most were critical of the service they had received from their GP 'They don't really pay attention to what we are saying and just write a prescription.' Their reported access to services depended largely on the presence of a friend or relative who could help navigate the system, as indicated by a 15-year-old Kosovan, 'I go with my uncle—he knows everything'.

It was clear that many of the young people required more information about services and how to access them. They stressed the importance of receiving information in their own language and suggested a 'website about health problems and issues for young people but in all languages'. However, their preference was face-to-face contact with someone who could provide information and advice. They suggested that this person should be based at their school, lending further support to the idea of a link worker that was proposed by the project.

Front-line staff and professionals echoed many of the same concerns articulated by young refugees and were aware that their service did not always meet the needs of refugees. A third felt they offered good services, and around a quarter said their service was fair. One in six said they thought the services they offered to young refugees were poor (Gosling 2000a). They cited communication and a lack of information as the main barriers to meeting the needs of young refugees. Less than a quarter had received any basic awareness training on refugee issues. A summary of the concerns raised by a range of service providers is outlined below.

Responses from service providers

- lack of provision to meet needs associated with isolation, loneliness, and boredom
- sexually active young refugee men not accessing information about safe sex
- concern about mental health of young refugees and lack of specialist provision
- vulnerability of unaccompanied minors, some as young as 14 years old, placed in adult accommodation, such as hostels
- lack of continuity of care from social workers
- intergenerational conflict while young refugees adapt to a different culture
- inadequacy of interpreting services
- confusion over roles and responsibilities within and between agencies with regards to the complex needs of young refugees
- concern about nutritional intake, particularly of unaccompanied minors
- lack of information/knowledge of specialist services, e.g. organisations offering support to victims of torture, refugee community organisations, or specialist refugee employment projects
- lack of coordination between different agencies, leading to problems making referrals and refugees falling 'between two stools'

- lack of school places for refugee children and lack of support for refugee children in schools (some children interviewed had waited up to eight months before they could find school placements)

The research identified a plethora of complex needs and the project faced the challenge of prioritising these needs and developing effective initiatives within the limitations of available resources. The research findings pointed towards the need for an inter-agency approach, training and information for front-line staff and professionals, health education and link workers to improve interagency working, sign posting and advocacy services for young refugees. Upon completion, the research report was widely disseminated across the HAZ partnership for information, comments, and suggestions (Gosling 2000b).

Action resulting from the research

By July 2001 the Young Refugee Project had employed three link workers, a health promotion specialist, a training and information officer, and a project coordinator. At the core of the project remain three key linked elements:

- inter-agency working
- improving access to services for young refugees
- the empowerment of young refugees

The link workers target discrete groups of young refugees: refugee children in schools, unaccompanied minors, and young refugees with disabilities or health problems. They assist young refugees to access services (health, education, social, leisure) and take on an advocacy role when access is blocked. The focus of their work is on providing information to the young refugees and supporting them to develop the skills and confidence to be able to access services independently in the future. Link Workers take on individual cases as well as running sessions with groups of young refugees. The team provides a telephone advice service to professionals, which often involves referring them to relevant services. For service providers who want to develop their knowledge further, a one-day training course has been developed.

The health promotion specialist works in partnership with refugee community organisations to pioneer peer education programs with young refugees through supplementary school and youth groups. Young refugees are trained on a range of health issues, including sexual health, so that they in turn can educate their peers. This is an empowering process for the peer educators who develop skills and become a valuable resource both for service providers and the youth in the community. There is also a parenting project for refugee families. A course to train refugees as health advocates or community health activists is in the planning stages.

The project team is in a position to identify where gaps in provision exist and provide leadership in the development of necessary programs. The team worked closely with Lambeth Child Health and Lambeth Social Services to establish a health clinic for unaccompanied minors. A qualified paediatrician assesses their medical needs, while the link worker deals with other issues that arise, such as finding a college place or registering with a GP.

These partnerships are facilitated by the existence of the inter-agency executive group who oversees the work of the project. The inter-agency executive group meets quarterly and is made up of representatives from both the statutory and voluntary sectors. The diversity represented within this group provides the project with an opportunity to solve problems, enabling it to take on board the different perspectives of the agencies represented. Examples of good practice are shared. Individual members of the executive group also have the responsibility to follow-up on issues identified and to work within their own agencies to influence change.

Discussion

The value of statutory and non-statutory, inter-disciplinary and multi-agency partnerships developed through HAZ is demonstrated by the outcomes of the study. The research findings have demonstrated that relatively modest initiatives like the LSL Young Refugee Project have the potential to serve as models of service coordination that could provide micro solutions to existing problems and be transferable to macro-level government policy within and even across departments. There is a need for improved and coordinated access to health, education, and social/community services for refugee children, young asylum seekers and their families. The role of link workers in providing two-way information service for young refugees and service providers alike is critical. The research process in itself has served to pave the way for a meaningful engagement of a wide variety of statutory health practitioners and voluntary/humanitarian agencies involved in supporting asylum seekers and refugees locally.

The two key requirements for effective coordination of services are information and communication. Data on asylum seekers and refugees is fraught with methodological and political problems internationally (Crisp 2000; Harrell-Bond et al. 1992) and locally. The research findings highlight the information gaps in terms of lack of data on numbers of asylum seekers and refugees and their addresses. These present major obstacles to effective service planning and funding. Communication and sharing of information between partner agencies is critical, but even at the level of individual agency or service providing institutions, routine data collection is not as straightforward as it may seem. For example, data on ethnicity did not previously appear in health service records as a matter of routine practice, either because health workers did not see the need to record details other than the service user's vital statistics and specific health complaint, or because the service user did not wish to provide that information. One of the new systems the HAZ instigated is the development and agreement of a Minimum Data Set (MDS) that should be collected and shared across the HAZ partnership. In theory, the value of an MDS in which service users' ethnicity and/or immigration status can be found would help service planning, funding, and impact evaluation. However, in practice, this may not help those serving asylum seekers and refugees as people are reluctant to disclose their immigration status (for understandable reasons), but data on language spoken would be useful as this has resource and planning implications, as the need for interpreters remains critical.

Young asylum seekers and refugees often find themselves in 'no win' situations. On the one hand, language barriers limit their access and use of services, while on the other children's quick acquisition of language may become a disadvantage to them as they assume the responsibility of interpreting for their parents at the risk of jeopardising their own educational and social development through school absenteeism and missed recreational/social opportunities. This may also jeopardise their parents'/carers' health and well-being, as adults who are reluctant to depend on their young children or relatives when seeking help with their own/private health and/or other needs may stay away from services. The ability to speak English is not in itself sufficient to enable refugee children and their families to access services. Two-way communication and mutual understanding requires more than just basic language proficiency. Implicit and/or explicit social and cultural attitudes come into play, and if the service provider has limited time, or knowledge or skills or inclination to assist asylum seekers, even those with the ability to communicate in English will remain excluded. The average consultation time of seven minutes per patient with a GP may not be sufficient time, particularly if the patient happens to be a child who depends on his/her carer to explain what the problem might be; and/or the carer requires an interpreter.

Previous studies had indicated that refugees may not consider health a priority for them (Aldous et al. 1999). Indeed, basic needs for food, shelter and employment/income with which to meet basic needs may be of more importance. Asylum seekers and refugees' top priorities are to put together their lives and livelihoods. There is a need to recognise existing community-based informal means of social support and welfare mechanisms that benefit those who are able to link up with them. For example, language and/or nationality-based refugee community organisations have long played a key role in promoting the health and well-being of asylum seekers and refugees by traditional support systems based on reciprocity and trust afforded by what Wilkinson (1996) calls 'social cohesion'. Their participation in and contribution to LSL's Young Refugee Project executive group is invaluable and would be expected to be measurable in terms of achieved health promotion targets through careful evaluation.

Also important are active measures to combat isolation, boredom, bullying and racial harassment. Refugee and/or migrant children carry multiple burdens of inter-generational and cross-cultural conflict and adaptation (Carballo et al. 1998). Girls may also experience added disadvantages on account of gender inequalities (Pittaway & Bartolomei 2001). This research did not allow for gender analysis, an area for further investigation.

The research has achieved its first and foremost aim of establishing inter-agency collaboration and multi-agency partnerships at the local level, essential elements of health promotion (Taket & White 2000). However, collaboration in itself is not going to be the 'acid test', when it comes to evaluation, because it is a health project and not a collaboration project. At the end of its three-year lifespan, if the project is unable to demonstrate that the health of asylum seekers and refugees has improved due to increased access to services—the project will have failed—in spite of producing better trained, skilled and as a result more empowered service providers.

The project continues to highlight the complex needs of young refugees, against a tide of negative media coverage and government policy, which continues to marginalise and alienate refugees and asylum seekers. This means that in addition to the barriers already mentioned, many young refugees and their families face discrimination and hostility, including from service providers themselves. However, a look behind the media portrayal reveals articulate, resilient young people willing and able to make a contribution to service development and wider society as a whole. The challenge for service providers is to create the opportunities for young refugees to express their views and experiences and to actively involve them, their parents and their communities while planning and delivering projects and services. One of the most important lessons learnt by the HAZ Young Refugee Project to date is that meaningful involvement of communities who are transient and distrusting of statutory bodies takes time to establish and can not always be achieved within the time frames of short-term funded projects.

Conclusion

The health and well-being of young asylum seekers and refugees in the UK presents complex and multifaceted sets of needs and priorities. What the LSL Young Refugee Project has achieved so far brings a ray of hope to what would otherwise be a situation of despair. The model of research involving multi-sectoral service providers and the users, in this case children and young people, is innovative and rewarding for all involved. More needs to be done by way of putting into practice knowledge and skills that already exist in the UK, so that young asylum seekers, and refugees and their families and communities may contribute productively to the health and well-being of their host communities, as well as their own.

Acknowledgments

The authors would like to thank Dr Ines Smyth (Oxfam, UK), Professor Sarah Cowley (King's College, London), Professor Lenore Manderson (University of Melbourne), Dr Anthony Tam (Southwark Primary Care Trust), Mr Ian Sandford and Ms Abigail Bennett (LSL Health Action Zone) for their constructive comments and suggestions on earlier drafts of this chapter. The generous support of LSL Health Action Zone (London) and the Henry R. Luce Program at Tufts University (Boston) is gratefully acknowledged. The views expressed in this chapter do not represent the above institutions.

Recommended reading

Bate, P. (2001) Synthesizing Research and Practice: Using the Action Research Approach in Health Care Settings, In Jones Finer C. & Lewando Hundt, G. (eds), *The Business of Research*, Blackwell, Oxford.

Steiner, N. (2000) *Arguing about asylum: the complexity of refugee debates in Europe*, St Martin's Press, New York.

Wilkinson R.G. (1996) *Unhealthy Societies: the afflictions of inequality*, Routledge, London.

References

Aldous, J., Bardsley, M., Daniel, R., Gair, R., Jacobson, B., Lowdell, C., Morgan, D. & Storkey, M. (1999) *Refugee Health in London: Key issues for Public Health*, Health of Londoners Project, East London and the City Health Authority, London.

Carballo, M., Divino, J.J. & Zeric, D. (1998) Migration and health in the European Union, *Tropical Medicine and International Health*, 3(12): 936–44.

Crisp, J. (2000) Who has counted the refugees? UNHCR and the politics of numbers, In S. Lubkemann, L. Minear & T. Weiss (eds), *Humanitarian Action: Social Science Connections* Occasional Paper #37, Watson Institute for International Studies, Brown University, Providence, pp. 33–62.

Dean, M. (1998) UK government announces first 'health action zones', *Lancet*, 351: 111.

Department of Health (1997) *Executive Letter (EL65), Health Action Zones: invitation to bid*, National Health Service Executive, London.

Gosling, R. (2000a) *The needs of young refugees in Lambeth, Southwark and Lewisham*, Lambeth, Southwark and Lewisham Health Action Zone Report, London.

Gosling, R. (2000b) *HAZ National Innovation Fund, Young Refugee Project Consultation Paper*, Community Health South London, London.

Harrel-Bond, B., Voutira, E. & Leopold, M. (1992) Counting the refugees: Gifts, givers, patrons and clients, *Journal of Refugee Studies*, 5 (3/4): 205–25.

Hewitt, R., Spicer, N. & Tooke, J. (2001) *Projects, participation and partnerships: An analysis of LSL HAZ activity*, Lambeth, Southwark and Lewisham Health Authority, Health Action Zone (HAZ) London.

Penz, P. (2000) Ethical Reflections on the Institution of Asylum, *Refuge*, 19(3): 44–53.

Petty, C. & Jareg, E. (1998) Conflict, poverty and family separation: The problem of institutional care, In Bracken, P. & Petty, C., (eds) *Rethinking the Trauma of War*, Save the Children Fund and Free Association Press, London and New York.

Refugee Council (1999) *In Exile*, Refugee Council, London.

Summerfield, D. (1997) The social, cultural and political dimensions of contemporary war, *Medicine, Conflict and Survival*, 13: 3–25.

Taket, A. & White, L. (2000) *Partnership and participation: decision making in the multi-agency setting*, John Wiley and Sons, Chichester.

UNHCR (1951) Convention relating to the status of refugees, UNHCR, Geneva.

UNHCR (1967) Protocol relation to the status of refugees, UNHCR, Geneva.

UNHCR (2002) Population Data Unit, March 2002, www.unhcr.ch, accessed on 29 July 2002.

Wilkinson R.G. (1996) *Unhealthy Societies: the afflictions of inequality*, Routledge, London.

12

Narratives of Forced Migration: Conducting Ethnographic Research with Somali Refugees in Australia

Celia McMichael

Introduction

This chapter discusses research with Somali women who have entered Australia through the refugee and humanitarian immigration program. Since the late 1970s, Somalia and other areas of the Horn of Africa have been wracked by violent conflict. Between December 1990 and January 1991, battle between government forces and clan-backed rebel groups resulted in the collapse of the twenty-one-year rule of the Somali dictator, General Siad Barre, and civil war erupted (Hashim 1997). Somalia has now been in a state of civil war for over ten years. The war, politically-induced famine, and drought have forced many people to flee their country. Hundreds of thousands of Somalis are in exile in Africa, in refugee camps, towns, and cities. Most must choose between the dangers of repatriation or remaining without citizenship in first countries of asylum; less than one per cent are accepted for resettlement in countries such as Australia (Hyndman 1999).

At the time of the 2001 Census of Population and Housing, there were 5007 Somali people living in Australia, of whom 48 per cent were female (Australian Bureau of Statistics 2002). The majority arrived after the eruption of the civil war, through Australia's refugee and humanitarian programs. Many women migrated to Australia through the 'Women at Risk' visa subclass, a category designated for women who do not have the protection of a male (Manderson et al. 1998; MRC North East 1999). The Somali-speaking community is one of the fastest-growing ethnic communities in Melbourne, increasing from 1391 in 1996 to 3226 in 2002. The research described in this chapter was conducted from April 2000 to August 2001, and took place in the northeastern region of Melbourne where there is a large Somali population.[1] This research explored the emotional well-being of Somali women in the context of war, displacement, and resettlement.

Field sites and researching refugees

Historically, anthropology has centred on conducting fieldwork with a view to producing an ethnography of a sociocultural space. Cultures were conceived as localised universes of meaning, with people and communities as their representative components. More recently, images of separate and contained worlds have been criticised as offering little more than a representational tool and ideology (James et al. 1997; Rapport & Dawson 1998). Migration and the movement of people unravels the notion of sociocultural places bound in space. There is no 'little Somalia' in Melbourne, no exclusive space where the Somali community can be found and researched. How, then, did I find a way to interact with Somali women and gain an ethnographic insight into their lives?

In April 2000 I started to volunteer at the Migrant Resource Centre Northeast (MRC), which provides direct services to a large number of Somali clients. This provided a concrete way in which to offer something to the women with whom I hoped to conduct research. The MRC is on a busy high street in a northeastern suburb of Melbourne. It sits at the beginning of a long stretch of community service offices and shops: a local office of the Department of Immigration and Multicultural and Indigenous Affairs (DIMIA), a Centrelink[2] office where people seek welfare payments, a regional government-funded emergency housing service, halal butchers, Iraqi and Turkish kebab shops, second-hand clothes and furniture stores, and the local market. The daily thoroughfare at the MRC is busy with 'newly-arrived migrants' most of whom have emigrated in the past six years from the former Yugoslavia, China, Iraq, and Somalia. The settlement team provides assistance with resettlement issues through a drop-in service, and an appointment system for people who present with more complex issues. Every week 20 to 25 Somali people, approximately two-thirds women, seek assistance with housing, health care, welfare benefits, and immigration advice.[3]

Omidian writes that, 'much field work is accomplished just by being in one place over time' (Omidian 1994 p. 155). Working with Malyun Ahmed, the Horn of Africa settlement support worker, I focused on resettlement issues and community development. Over the first few months, Malyun taught me the basics of settlement support casework: how to assist with Office of Housing applications, where to refer people for material aid such as second-hand furniture, what kind of no-interest-loan schemes[4] are available in the region, how to secure government rebates for utility service bills, how to nominate a family for refugee visas, and how to use the Telephone Interpreting Service. Soon I gained enough confidence to help 'clients' through the complex maze of social services.

The beginning of my voluntary work at the MRC marks the start of the research phase:

> This is a new world for me, but I am learning slowly. Sounds I hear repeated in language—haye (yes), mia (no), seeye tata (how are you?), wa fia anahai (I'm fine). I am struck by the confused contrasts in my mind. There is a too-easy romantic picture of Somali women as strong and colourful nomads making their way in a foreign city; the rhythms of the language, the swish of women's henna-dyed hands when they touch in expressive gestures, the colours and weave of cloth readjusted and folded around faces. Then sometimes I feel so sad. Stories are hard to hear. It is difficult to read the brutal details written in visa applications of being forced to watch family being raped and killed at gunpoint, the pain of leaving behind one's home and life, the hardship of flight and living in refugee camps.
>
> Field note excerpt, May 2000

As I continued to work at the MRC, I became accustomed to spending time with the women. They were no longer mysterious figures defined by the war and the associated suffering, but real women with real lives. I started to understand something of different Somali women's histories, became aware of the hardship and trauma of war that many women suffered, assisted with resettlement, and began to appreciate women's resilience and strength. In turn, women came to recognise and know me.

During lunch breaks, Malyun and I clarified my intended research. I explained my interest in disrupted lives, community and depression, and she told me about the experience and prevalence of sadness, loneliness, and depression among Somali women. Malyun was not only enthusiastic and supportive of the research, but wanted to be involved. As I discuss below, Malyun played a key role in the research process, namely interpreting, assisting with the practicalities of the research, analysis of the interviews, and support. We began to spend time visiting Somali women's homes, and Malyun invited me to events so that I could be involved socially with women outside of the MRC setting.

One evening, soon after I began working with Malyun, we visited Amina at her Office of Housing low-rise property—a ground floor flat in a block of six built from weathered red-brick. She was at home with her children, feeding them rice while the television played. The living room floor was covered with large Persian carpets. A wooden cabinet was pushed against one wall and decorated with plastic flowers, a painted china tea-set, and plates inscribed with Islamic texts; the other walls were adorned with prints covered with ornate gold Islamic calligraphy. The smell of sweet-cardamom tea and incense hung in the air. We gathered in the kitchen to make *sambuusas*. Amina spoke on the phone while she made the pastry, Malyun crouched down to pound a paste from onion and garlic with a wooden pestle and mortar, and I stirred the meat and vegetables in hot oil while Amina's children clamoured and pulled my clothes and necklace. Then we formed an assembly line, rolling out pastry and filling it with halal mince and vegetables and deep-frying the golden pastries. Malyun and Amina spoke in Somali, their conversation inter-jected with the occasional English terms of '3-bedroom house' or 'the problem is': they were talking about housing troubles. After we finished cooking, Amina got me to try on a silk dress and some beautiful orange cloth, shot with gold thread, that she wanted me to wear at an upcoming party. They laughed when they saw me, but thought that the clothes looked better than my 'Australian' ones. Shared times, such as this, allowed women to become accustomed to me. Malyun agreed that as women grew used to my presence, they felt more comfortable talking with us.

The section above gives some flavour of the environment in which the research process took place. For a diasporic community such as the Somali in Melbourne, however, a focus on the immediate fieldsite obscures the dispersed domains of transnational relationships, displacement and migra-tion. Conversations with women included talk of their homeland, ongoing relationships with family overseas, refugee camps and exile, and compari-son of immediate lifeworlds with nostalgic recollection of Somalia. In this research the *field* was not confined to the tangible parameters of an imme-diate setting, and accordingly I focused on relations, movement, and memory as much as situated community and spatial location.

Research methods

'Participant' observation

Conventional anthropology has dictated that participating in a commu-nity is integral to understanding the meanings and experiences that con-stitute a cultural world. Abu-Lughod (1986 p. 22) argues that living in the social world that one is studying allows the researcher to grasp more immediately how social worlds work and how members understand it. Among other things, I went to women's gatherings and celebrations, shared meals in people's homes, attended information sessions for Somalis, and helped women negotiate Office of Housing applications.

> Yesterday I spent hours in a room full of women, sitting amidst dynamic and raucous talk and laughter, but I was sad that I didn't understand the meaning of their words. So I tried to be patient, sat back and drank the endless cups of too-sweet milky tea, and ate a plate piled high with pasta and meat. I played with the kids who looked at me with curious eyes, meanwhile Fatuma's baby dribbled milk down my top. Sometimes I found myself being distracted by the background noise of television. I watched women come and go, Hakimo's son came in, unrolled the prayer mat, and carried out his prayers, children careered between outstretched arms, the women talked and laughed.
>
> Field note excerpt, November 2000

Participation in community and social activities brought richness to my understanding of women's lives. Working in social settings of displacement and resettlement, however, invites questioning of anthropological concepts of *participant* observation. A significant barrier to participant observation is that, as refugees, Somali women's lifeworlds extend to spaces and experiences beyond the reach of ethnographic observation or participation. I could never share the traumas and hardships of civil war, displacement, and resettlement, be subject to racism, or live in the knowledge that I could not return to my country and life as it was before war. One evening, Ismahan asked me about my family, and I explained that they live overseas. She responded:

> If you haven't got a family here, then you still feel distressed because they are not around you, there is no person that is there for you in the country. And that is also why many Somali women get depressed. Imagine, though, if you face civil war, or your sister or family is dead from the war, or you lost your family. Women feel this stress. You left places by choice and you can go back some day, but with a civil war it is different. This one is without choice.

Ismahan suggests that while I could empathise with Somali women's experience of family separation, I could never have a participatory understanding. My *participant* observation was limited by the reality that refugees are displaced; many aspects of their lives can never be shared by a researcher from a non-refugee background.

The interview process

One afternoon Malyun and I dropped by Isir's house to see if she had time to speak with us. She welcomed us in to her living room. While we sipped cups of tea, Malyun explained the themes of the research. Isir carefully curled her feet up underneath herself on the chair, checked that the tape recorder was running, and began by saying:

> My story is worth the story of ten women. Life was good until 1990. From the beginning of the civil war that went from 1991 to 1998, all I can say is that I have died...

Isir went on to describe her nostalgic memories of Somalia, the eruption of the civil war, terrible conditions of exile in Ethiopia, separation from her family following the acceptance of their Australian refugee visa applications, and finally resettlement in Melbourne. She has five children, but her youngest remains in Ethiopia due to visa complications. Isir suffers from depression and has been prescribed antidepressants. The narratives that emerged in this interview and others were a significant source for learning about and understanding women's lives.

The interviews took place over eleven months, from September 2000 to July 2001, and were conducted with forty-two women. Women's ages ranged from 19 to 65, and their socio-economic backgrounds and contemporary circumstances varied. Burgess (1991: 45) argues that in ethnographic research, access to a community or group of people depends on the relationships that are established between the researcher and the researched. As an emerging migrant community, Somalis have been the target of a number of research projects and are tired of being researched (Nsubage-Kyobe & Dimock 2000). I was therefore unwilling to recruit women through impersonal 'random sample' techniques. The selection of women to participate in the study centred around Malyun's extensive network of friendships and acquaintances, the relationships I formed with women through my work at the MRC, and women's willingness to participate.

Due to the time constraints of doctoral research, I was unable to learn sufficient Somali language to converse and carry out interviews. My rudimentary knowledge of Somali and the limited English language of many Somali women meant that I relied on Malyun to interpret for thirty-three of the interviews. Malyun did not act merely as an interpreter, however, but also as a key informant and co-researcher. She was able to pursue sensitively issues that I might have left, we discussed research themes, and we talked about issues that I felt I hadn't grasped. I did not *use* an interpreter, but *worked with* an interpreter, informant, and co-researcher.

Interviews were conducted in women's homes, their own or a friend's. Before beginning interviews, Malyun asked whether I could tape-record or take notes during interviews. A few women preferred that I take notes, but some later insisted that I put on the tape recorder in order that everything would be documented. During interviews, I was sometimes asked to stop recording if issues were too private or volatile to be documented, as was sometimes the case with respect to sexual relations, dissatisfaction with the current immigration program, or community politics. This negotiation around recording suggests that women had a keen awareness of the research process, a sense of talking to a wider audience, and an understanding of issues of consent in that *they* decided what aspects of their lives to share.

I began the interviews by asking an initial question such as, 'Can you tell me your story of coming to live in Melbourne?' or 'Can you talk about your life in Somalia?' Many women talked without hesitation, but if women became uncertain about the course of their narratives, then I prompted them with questions to maintain the flow of conversation. The largely non-directive nature of conversations allowed women to form their accounts in their own words, around themes and events that they deemed most interesting and central to their lives. Interviews lasted from between half an hour to six hours, and some women spoke with us on more than one occasion. At the end of interviews, I asked women if they had anything to add or any questions to ask. Many women were curious about my life—whether I had a partner, how large my family was—and their questions were sometimes about 'private' issues such as sex and love. Others asked about the research process. I tried to answer questions openly, often resulting in funny situations as women teased me, for example, about being so old and still not having children. A number of women simply thanked us for listening.

While the majority of interviews took place with individual women, on several occasions we spoke with a number of women at a time. These group discussions were not focus group discussions with explicit methodological aims (Bernard 1994; Dawson et al. 1993; Hudelson 1994; Patton 1990); rather, they were haphazard, the product of circumstance. Sometimes we went to a woman's house and the too-many pairs of shoes at the door and sounds of talking gave away the presence of more women than anticipated, and so we took the opportunity to have a group discussion. The composition of groups changed as people arrived and left the house, went to the kitchen to prepare food, or unrolled mats on the floor and began prayers. Impromptu group discussions encouraged women to talk about their experiences. Women felt comfortable and open, particularly as the friendships within the groups were established. Further, I avoided the logistical arrangements of recruitment, finding an appropriate time and place, and anxiety that people would not show up. The emergence of differing views, however, was especially fruitful and group discussions provided an opportunity for women to tease out divergencies in their experiences.

Listening to narratives

> Narrative is a form in which experience is represented and recounted, in which events are presented as having a meaningful and coherent order, in which activities and events are described along with the experiences associated with them and the significance that lends them their sense for the persons involved.
>
> (Good 1994: 139)

When people apply for refugee and humanitarian application visas for Australia, they are required to write about their experiences of persecution, how they left their country, and what they think will happen to them if they return. If they are selected, they go through a rigorous interviewing process to ascertain the truthfulness of their accounts. Narrative research is very different from this process. It allows for changes and multiple versions in meaning, experiences, interpretation, and explanations (Bruner 1987; Kirkman 1997). Narrative frameworks are particularly relevant for interpreting the disrupted experience of exile and resettlement as they allow people to draw together disparate aspects of experience into a coherent whole (Becker 1997 p. 25). The collection of narratives was not a tool that I used to produce an account of the *truth* of women's experience (Kirkman & Rosenthal 1999 pp. 19–20; Scheper-Hughes 1992; Wikan 1996). Rather, I explored how women ascribe meaning and order to their lives. In their narratives, images emerged of nostalgic memory for homeland, the civil war, fleeing Somalia, living in refugee camps and other countries of asylum, their expectations and the realities of life in Australia, and imagined futures. Women could have told their stories differently, or focused on different events or meanings. The important thing is that their stories were meaningful at the time of telling.

Refugees are often regarded as generic figures, represented as floods, waves and streams rather than as individuals with different lives. This leads to generalisations that mask the humanity and varying experiences of individuals, and depict an image of refugees as an amorphous *other*. Through narrative research, it has been possible to retain the integrity and diversity of women's accounts of displacement and resettlement. Women had different understandings, for example, of the refugee label, diverse experiences of *community* following resettlement, and varied accounts of the causes of their emotional distress. When talking about community relations in Melbourne, one woman said:

> After the war, for the first time the people lost trust in each other. Now there is tribalism, everyone has to go to his own tribe . . . everyone is feeling that [distrust] inside. I don't like the people that killed my brother, even though they are just a clan ... I don't feel that nice about them. As a human, if I saw them I would just say hi, but inside my heart I don't feel like having a friend from that tribe.

By contrast, another woman said:

> For me, clan is not important. I think we are all Somali. We are all the same. I don't think about my clan. To think about clan leads to bad things. It is because of clans that there is fighting in Somalia. In Australia now, clan is not important. We have seen the damage it can do and now we are all just equal. There are no higher or lower people here, everyone is just the same.

This diversity resonates with the project of 'writing against culture' that retains individual voices as an alternative to essentialist claims about cultures or groups of people (Abu-Lughod 1986; Comaroff & Comaroff 1992). From this view, the thing to underscore in ethnography and other social representation is fluidity, the uneven social and political conditions of people's lives, and divergent experiences and memories, and then to map out alternative meanings and moralities. Yet as I listened for diversity, I was also struck by the thematic convergence in women's narratives. There were many instances where women presented consensual accounts of their histories and contemporary lives: widespread nostalgia for Somalia, and similarities in the hardships faced in Melbourne, are cases in point.

How, then, to make sense of the narratives that I heard? Women's narratives entailed both the coherence of shared themes, and diversity within individual narratives. Jean and John Comaroff (1992) write, 'with a sufficiently supple view of culture, we may begin to understand why social life everywhere appears dualistic, simultaneously ordered and disorderly' (p. 30). It is unnecessary to make a choice between the modernist perspective that searches out unity within 'culture', and a postmodern perspective in which the world is a partially integrated mosaic of narratives, images, and contested signifying practices. Women's narratives were not ordered and constant; they contained both a measure of predictability, and the uncertain, indeterminate, and creative.

Silence

The discussion above has explored how women gave voice to their experiences. Yet it is also important to think about the significance of silences; what women did not to say, and what they could not say (Poland & Pederson 1998). In neo-positivist methodology, the researcher's role is to discover that which is hidden, deemed irrelevant, or kept secret, and to illuminate these discoveries with scientific scrutiny (Mitchell 1991: 97). A classic text on ethnographic interviewing states explicitly that a principle of interviewing is to 'keep informants talking' (Spradley 1979: 8). During this research, many women's narratives were punctuated by silence, particularly around the civil war and refugee camps. However, I did not seek to draw out the 'data' behind silence and determine what was left unsaid, but respected women's right to decide whether, and to what extent, to relate experiences.

Studies of popular memory and history suggest that narratives, and the silences and omissions they entail, play an essential part in the construction of people's past (Malkki 1995; Swedenburg 1995; Wright 1985). In this research, many women crystallised a nostalgic view of a past moral order, tradition, community, and culture. Daily life in Somalia was recalled as infused with solidarity, sharing, and support:

> The best thing that I remember is that after people woke up, they went outside to see everybody. In Somalia, most of the houses have a small seat at the front and all the neighbours would sit outside in groups and have a cup of tea and chat. When that chatting finishes, around sunset, we could put on nice clothes and go outside without worrying that someone might hurt you. There was a sense of freedom, a sense of community, a sense of togetherness, and chatting, and knowing all the neighbours. We would all know about each other's business. That was the best thing.

I heard similar narratives of community, connectedness and social support, time and time again. In contrast, the silence around hardships in Somalia was striking. Few women mentioned social inequality, hardship, or personal experiences of sadness in Somalia. The refrain, 'in Somalia, life was good', was constant. Silence and omission was a way to bring the force of imagination into narratives, a way to rework and revise the past. This configuration of life in Somalia provided a social and moral framework with which to compare the exigencies of everyday life in Melbourne.

There were also silences around specific experiences. Some women chose not to speak of the war, swiftly moving from narratives of pre-war Somalia to arrival in Australia. Others described the war as a series of events and processes entailing generalised and abstract details, without emotional edge:

They gathered everyone, they had kept two men alive and they killed everyone else. Most of the men from the south had either died or had to run away.
They had only two men remaining alive. They gathered all the women and
children in a clinic. Some of the women's husbands were lying there dead.
When the women gathered, they realised they were widows. Their innocent
husbands had just been walking around, and now they were dead. They did
not dare to look at their bodies, because if they looked at them and the militia said 'is that your husband?', then they would have to say 'no', or else the
militia would know that they weren't Isaak.[5] The women didn't even dare to
cry. They just looked around quickly and said they didn't see their husband.
The militia brought the two men and they started cutting them into pieces in
front of us. The guns had a knife on the ends, and they took their eyes out
with the knives. I vomited. I was sick. I vomited.

Narratives such as this were often presented with startling detachment,
the details of personal lives taken only to the point of enunciating facts.
Yet even with verbal silence around emotional experience, the sadness,
trauma, and memory of terror was often manifest as tears, or visible efforts
to reorder memory into a less disturbing sequence. I accepted silences
within narratives out of respect for women's integrity. On further reflection, I also understood silence as a form of communication that enabled
women to construct their narratives in meaningful and acceptable ways.

Ethical issues

At the very least, we have to confront the complexities of our relations to our
subject, texts, and audiences—especially because the impact of our work is
never fully foreseeable. This not only demands a serious regard, once again, for
contexts, our own as much as those we study. It also calls for a careful consideration of the real implications of what we do, a consideration that must go far
beyond the now routine recognition that our writings are potential instruments of 'othering'.

(Comaroff & Comaroff 1992 p. 12)

Social research should benefit the population or group of people on
whom it focuses. The World Health Organisation (WHO) states that one
way to ensure that participants benefit from research is to involve direct
service groups from the outset (World Health Organisation 1999).
Through our work at the MRC, Malyun and I were able to respond
actively to some of the themes and concerns raised in interviews. When
women talked about specific resettlement concerns, such as housing and

immigration, we offered assistance in the capacity of settlement case-workers. We also used the research findings in community development programs that aim to strengthen social networks and address resettlement problems. Malyun organised and ran a number information sessions and group discussions for Somali women on specific themes, including parenting, emotional well-being, and discrimination. We organised social outings, such as picnics and lunches, in response to women's sense of isolation and loneliness.

I also hoped that the interviews could be an opportunity for women to give voice to their experiences in a safe and supportive environment. Psychiatric literature suggests that for survivors of torture and trauma, recounting such experiences can provide effective symptomatic relief (Young 1993). However, others do not view voiced elaboration of emotional worlds as a cathartic process, but as one that forces the person to continually return to an awareness of their depression, so that 'they keep turning it over, helplessly' (Kristeva 1987). Some clinical research suggests that the retrospective questioning that is characteristic of psychiatric therapy causes post-traumatic symptoms to intensify (Boehnlein et al. 1985). Given this uncertainty around the benefit of recounting traumatic experience, I did not push women to talk about distressing themes or events. Many women welcomed the opportunity to talk about difficult experiences, others avoided distressing events entirely, and others still spoke of the war in a tone that sounded as if they were compelled to do so but gained neither benefit nor relief. It was important to offer women the chance to talk about trauma and war; the decision to do so was theirs.

Conducting social research always involves ethical issues and dilemmas in relation to study groups and populations; however, little has been written about the impact of the research process for the researcher. Omidian (1994) writes, 'work with refugees has special problems for the researcher because of the trauma that population has experienced' (p. 171). There were many times during the research when I was distressed by stories of war, loss, death, and struggles with resettlement in Melbourne. I found that I was often thinking about the stories I heard, having nightmares, and imagining myself in the same situations. I sometimes cried during interviews and later, while transcribing interviews and notes, and felt guilty that there was nothing I could do to change women's histories of enduring war and violence. This experience is not uncommon among people who work with refugees (Dunn 1991; Omidian 1994).

There were a number of ways that I reduced my anxiety and distress. Writing field notes was a good way to express my reactions. I sometimes talked about interviews with my partner, supervisor, and Malyun, trusted people who allowed me to 'debrief'. Ongoing involvement in work at the MRC warded off feelings of helplessness, as Malyun and I worked to ensure that the research has applied benefit. Participation in positive aspects of Somali women's lives helped to maintain perspective, as their lives were shown to be much broader than the remembered horror of war. Further, women's narratives included accounts of nostalgic memory, resilience, times of enjoyment and happiness, and good things about countries of resettlement, and these aspects of their lives were more audible when I was not emotionally strained.

Conclusion

The research described above did not revolve around a determination to uncover the truth, but on a willingness to allow women to direct the course of the research and interviews. I did not view myself as an anthropologist trying to piece together a cultural puzzle about *refugee* experience through the collection and analysis of data. Like Malkki (1995), I found that 'sometimes what is called for is not an 'investigator' at all, but an attentive listener' (p. 51). Much of the research was accomplished by spending time with women, listening to stories and the things that women deemed as important, and understanding that women are not simply refugees but people with diverse histories and lives. Finally, richness was brought to the research through ongoing work at the MRC and collaborating with Malyun.

Recommended reading

James, A., Hockey, J. & Dawson, A. (1997) *After Writing Culture*, Routledge, London.

Omidian, P. (1994) Life Out of Context: Recording Afghan Refugees' Stories, In eds, Camino, L., Krulfeld, R., Boone, M. & DeVoe, P. (eds), *Reconstructing Lives, Recapturing Meaning: Refugee identity, gender, culture*, Gordon and Breach Science Publishers, Basel.

Poland, B. & Pederson, A. (1998) Reading Between the Lines: interpreting silences in qualitative research, *Qualitative Inquiry*, 4(2): 293–316

References

ABS (2002) Australian Demographic Statistics, http://www.abs.gov.au.

Abu-Lughod, L. (1986) *Veiled Sentiments: Honor and poetry in a Bedouin society*, University of California Press, Los Angeles and London.

Becker, G. (1997) *Disrupted Lives*, University of California Press, California.

Bernard, H.R. (1994) *Research Methods in Anthropology*, Sage Publications, London.

Boehnlein, J.K., Kinzie, J.D., Rath, B. & Fleck, J. (1985) One-year follow-up study of posttraumatic stress disorder among survivors in Southeast Asian refugees, *American Journal of Psychiatry*, 142: 956–9.

Bruner, J. (1987) Life as Narrative, *Social Research*, 54: 11–32.

Burgess, R. (1991) Access in educational settings, In Shaffir, W.B. & Stebbins, R.A. (eds), *Experiencing Fieldwork*, Sage Publications, London.

Comaroff, J. & Comaroff, J. (1992) *Ethnography and the Historical Imagination*, Westview Press, Colorado.

Dawson, S., Manderson, L. & Tallo, V. (1993) *A Manual for Focus Groups*, International Nutrition Foundation for Developing Countries, Boston.

Dunn, L. (1991) Research Alert! Qualitative research may be hazardous to your health! *Qualitative Health Research*, 1(3): 388–92.

Good, B. (1994) *Medicine, Rationality and Experience*, Cambridge University Press, Cambridge.

Hashim, A.B. (1997) *The Fallen State: Dissonance, Dictatorship and Death in Somalia*, University Press of America, Maryland and Oxford.

Hudelson, P. (1994) *Qualitative Research for Health Programmes*, Division of Mental Health, World Health Organisation, Geneva.

Hyndman, J. (1999) A post-cold war geography of forced migration in Kenya and Somalia, *Professional Geographer*, 51(1): 104–14.

James, A., Hockey, J. & Dawson, A. (1997) Introduction: the road from Santa Fe, In James, A., Hockey, J. & Dawson, A. (eds), *After Writing Culture*, Routledge, London.

Kirkman, M. (1997) Plots and disruptions: narratives, infertility, and women's lives, unpublished doctoral dissertation, La Trobe University, Victoria, Australia.

Kirkman, M. & Rosenthal, D. (1999) Representations of Reproductive Technology in Women's Narratives of Infertility, *Women & Health*, 29(2): 17–35.

Kristeva, J. (1987) *Black Sun: Depression and Melancholia*, Columbia University Press, USA.

Malkki, L. (1995) *Purity and Exile*, University of Chicago Press, Chicago.

Manderson, L., Kelaher, K., Williams, G. & Shannon, C. (1998) The politics of community: Negotiation and consultation in research on women's health, *Human Organization*, 57(2): 222–39.

Mitchell, R.G. (1991) Secrecy and disclosure in Fieldwork, In Shaffir, W.B. & Stebbins, R.A. (eds), *Experiencing Fieldwork*, Sage Publications, London.

MRC North East (1999) MRC Annual Report 1999, North East Migrant Resource Centre, Melbourne.

Nsubage-Kyobe, A. & Dimock, L. (2000) *African Communities and Settlement Services in Victoria: Towards Best Practice Service Delivery Models*, Department of Immigration and Multicultural and Indigenous Affairs, Australia.

Omidian, P. (1994) Life Out of Context: Recording Afghan Refugees' Stories, In Camino, L., Krulfeld, R., Boone, M. & DeVoe, P. (eds), *Reconstructing Lives, Recapturing Meaning: Refugee identity, gender, culture*, Gordon and Breach Science Publishers, Basel.

Patton, M. (1990) *Qualitative Evaluation and Research Methods*, Sage, London and New Delhi.

Poland, B. & Pederson, A. (1998) Reading Between the Lines: interpreting silences in qualitative research, *Qualitative Inquiry*, 4(2): 293-316.

Rapport, N. & Dawson, A. (1998) The Topic and The Book, In Rapport, N. & Dawson, A. (eds), *Migrants of Identity*, Berg, Oxford and New York.

Scheper-Hughes, N. (1992) *Death Without Weeping*, University of California Press, Berkeley.

Spradley, J.P. (1979) *The Ethnographic Interview*, Harcourt Brace Jovanovich, Fort Worth, TX.

Swedenburg, T. (1995) *Memories of Revolt: The 1936-39 Rebellion and the Palestinian National Past*, University of Minnesota Press, Minneapolis.

Wikan, U. (1996) *Tomorrow, God Willing: self-made destinies in Cairo*, Chicago University Press, Chicago & London.

World Health Organisation (1999) *Putting Women First: Ethical and Safety Recommendations for Research on Domestic Violence Against Women*, World Health Organisation, Geneva, pp. 1-13.

Wright, P. (1985) *On living in an Old Country: the national past in contemporary Britain*, Verso, London.

Young, A. (1993) A description of how ideology shapes knowledge of a mental disorder (Posttraumatic Stress Disorder), In Lindenbaum, S. & Lock, M. (eds), *Knowledge, Power and practice: the anthropology of medicine and everyday life*, University of California Press, London.

Notes

1   This research was carried out as part of a doctoral program at the University of Melbourne.

2   'Centrelink' is a government service that manages social security/welfare payments in Australia.

3   This data is based on a twelve-month period in 2000–01 and is generated from the MRC client database.

4   NILS are primarily available for white-goods such as washing machines and refrigerators, and educational courses.

5   Isaak is the name of one of the Somali clans.

13

From Case Studies to Casework: Ethics and Obligations in Research with Refugee Women

Pascale Allotey and Lenore Manderson

Introduction

The vulnerability of refugees and resettled communities described in the preceding chapters makes them an important focus of research in bio-medical, public health, and social sciences. The vulnerability creates an unequal relationship in the research process that has been highlighted in feminist research. In 1981 Helen Roberts and colleagues suggested that feminist praxis demanded an ethical relationship between women researchers and their study participants. Women, they argued, are more likely to be aware of and uncomfortable with the inherently unequal relationships between researcher and participants, and seek to minimise inequality by establishing research-based friendships, even if these are somewhat pragmatic and opportunistic, and to maintain them over time. The renegotiation of conventional power relations of researcher and subject has epistemological, technical, and personal implications. Method-ological approaches shape social relationships in different ways. Formal structured interviews, for example, maintain distance between inter-viewer and respondent that is impossible in unstructured interviews, within which the balance of power and decision making shifts from inter-viewer/researcher to interviewee/participant. Participant-observation rather than survey-style methods enables the researcher to establish a close relationship with study participants beyond the conventional expression of 'rapport' and sympathy, resulting in a grounded and holistic, context-rich, understanding of participants' lives. In turn, it demands both emotional and ethical responsibility. The apparent differences in gender styles contribute to differences in the production of knowledge: the pre-eminence of epidemiological survey-style research among doctors (predominantly male), for example, contrasts with the marked preference for qualitative research by nurses.

Concurrent with discussions of power differences in the conduct of research that has occurred over the past two decades is the increasing attention that has been given to other factors that produce unequal relationships between researchers and research communities. In response to representations from researched communities who have managed to voice their concern regarding their objectification in the research process, increasing attention has been paid to the ethical obligations of researchers, the role of research participants as collaborators and their need for tangible returns from researchers. Consequently, the ethical guidelines of professional associations and institutional ethics committees have drawn attention to the need to minimise structural inequalities, not simply the procedural honouring of ethical principles (such as informed consent), but also with respect to everyday conduct, sensitivity, care, partnership, and empowerment. Notions of risk, benefit and harm are implicit in these principles. The ethical obligations to communities, and the implications of this for practice, have been discussed as they relate to work with indigenous communities, although how formal ethical obligations translate into everyday social relations, within both a research context and a wider social and political context, has received less attention (Manderson et al. 2001; Manderson & Wilson 1998). It has been the politically charged relationship between researchers and communities that resulted in the focus on indigenous Australians, but the issues that arise in this context are ones that occur more broadly and are partly reflected in resource differences between the researchers and communities with whom researchers conventionally work.

In this chapter, we explore the ethical issues that developed within and derived from our work with refugee women. The paper foregrounds the personal and professional demands of any research, but particularly the imperative when working with people who have limited contact with the service sector, for whom the researcher represents an avenue of practical assistance and redress. The issues that we examine are grounded in case studies from our work with humanitarian settlers from Sahel Africa and the Middle East (SAME), now living in Melbourne, Australia. The cases have been constructed based on data from the study to highlight the relevant issues and at the same time to obscure the identities of the participants. Pseudonyms have been used for the same reason.

The study

Approximately 87,000 women from SAME countries are resident in Australia, entering the country either as migrants or humanitarian settlers or refugees (Australian Bureau of Statistics 1996). Newly arrived women from countries such as Ethiopia, Eritrea, Somalia and Sudan, with longer-term immigrants from Egypt, Lebanon, and Syria, make up a significant proportion of visible minority groups in Australia because of skin colour and preference for traditional clothing and veils. Their reproductive health is of particular concern for a number of reasons including high fertility rates, cultural practices such as various degrees of female genital excision and lack of engagement with reproductive health services. Our study aimed to investigate reproductive health issues and indicators that affect the general well-being of these migrant and refugee women.

Health problems derive from specific cultural beliefs or practices, but also as a result of socio-economic status prior to and after migration, and to illness, infection and trauma in countries of origin and in transition. There is a higher incidence of infectious diseases among refugees from developing countries (see Biggs and Skull), and women have pre-existing nutritional, gynaecological, and/or mental health problems (see Kaplan p. 104). Many women have a high risk for poor obstetric outcomes, in part as a result of greater parity, and higher prevalence of anaemia, urinary tract infections, and sexually transmissible infections largely as a result of sexual abuse and exploitation. Further, in many of the SAME countries, health education and health promotion activities are uncommon, women's health is not discussed publicly and the education of women is not encouraged. These factors influence women's understanding of their health, and their use of various services in Australia. The gender of the provider, the availability of translators, fear of hospitalisation, and concerns about interventions and how they could affect the integrity of the body all influence women's willingness to present for care and to accept treatment advice.

The research was a qualitative study that was developed with the advice and support of a Community Advisory Group, which included representatives from a number of community agencies and service providers, as well as individuals. The group facilitated communication between researchers, the SAME communities, and service providers thereby enhancing participation, ownership, and relevance of the study. Through regular meetings, the group functioned to inform the research process, disseminate information, and provide advocacy for policy and programs for the target population. Some 255 women were interviewed and followed up for the three-year duration of the study. The Sahel African women were from Somalia, Ethiopia, Eritrea, Sudan, Chad, Nigeria, and Ghana; the Middle

Eastern women from Saudi Arabia, Egypt, Lebanon, Iraq, Iran, and Palestine. Data were collected with a combination of qualitative (focus groups, in-depth interviews and narratives) and quantitative research techniques (measurement of quality of life and health status).

The study had strong links with the Family and Reproductive Rights Education Program (FARREP) of the Victorian Department of Human Services, the state initiative of the National Education Program on Female Genital Mutilation. A major strength of the study was the employment of bicultural workers for the recruitment of participants and assistance in data collection from women from the refugee communities. Two research assistants were employed, one from Egypt to work with the Middle Eastern women and one from Eritrea to work with the Sahel African women. Both women had professional backgrounds in social and community development work with several years of experience as bicultural workers.

Working with bicultural workers

Bicultural workers are a heterogeneous category of workers in terms of age, educational backgrounds, and motivation for employment (Tribe 1999) and are usually from refugee and migrant communities. Many use it as an opportunity to enter the workforce and others as an opportunity to help their communities. Their skill levels vary ranging from those who are highly qualified but are unable to get their degrees recognised in Australia to those with little to no formal qualifications, but an exceptional ability to advocate for members of their community.

The use of bicultural workers is the preferred model of service provision to communities from refugee and culturally and linguistically diverse backgrounds (Kelaher & Manderson 2000). Their role is central to bridging the gap between the host society and the migrant communities from which they originate. This role has been identified as effective in achieving health outcomes (Corkery et al. 1997) and responsive to women's needs, providing a role of mediation between existing health services that may not be well understood and perceived as culturally inappropriate for many women (Manderson & Allotey 2003a). Difficulties have arisen however, when some bicultural workers or clients will only engage with those who share their political view or ethnic backgrounds. There have also been complaints about inaccurate translations (Riddick 1998; Tribe 1999). Bicultural workers are often employed on a casual basis, which precludes security in employment, a career structure, and any real authority on which to advocate for women from their communities. Furthermore, it remains unclear if the workers are responsible to the community and therefore the client or to the employing service provider and organisation (Musser-Granski & Carillo 1997).

An important issue was highlighted in our work with bicultural workers who were in the sample of women interviewed. A significant proportion of refugee women (including those who are employed as bicultural workers) have undergone traumatic experiences in the conflict and post conflict situations. The potential trauma for bicultural workers as they tried to support patients, many of whom were working through the resolution of past experiences, was seldom recognised by the agencies with which they were employed. The following provides a description of one woman's experience.

> Can you understand what it is like to feel too guilty to be miserable when I have a bad day? I have a lot to be thankful for. I live in a safe country, I have a job, I speak English and I can mostly understand what is going on and I can stand up for myself. I am also in a position to do something for my community and many many people are in a bad way, they are really suffering. I work with these women and I know what they are going through. They talk about things, about experiences that I have had but have never spoken about, I have been where they have been myself and I know how it hurts. But somehow I have been lucky. I don't feel lucky all the time and I know that when I don't, all I have to do is go to work and there is someone I have to go and see who is worse than me. But still it can be really hard not to just scream at the world or just hide away on some days. Some of it is in the work, sometimes it's just life. But I always think, don't be stupid, what do I have to complain about; I don't have the luxury to feel miserable because I am blessed. I have to keep going. Things could be much worse.

Despite the heterogeneity of backgrounds and the apparent central role for practice in multicultural settings, very little research has been conducted with bicultural workers to explore models of best practice to maximise outcomes for patients, service providers, and the workers themselves. Collectively, bicultural workers present an impressive level of resilience that could provide an important resource for public health, and there is clearly a need for research that identifies the obstacles to their effective practice.

From case studies to casework

Our research assistants, both also bicultural workers, assisted in the collection of data for the construction of case studies. They met with women and other members of their families professionally and informally. Women saw them as a resource, both because of their knowledge of community and state resources and systems and because of women's expectations of the return from their participation in the research. Communication between the research assistants and research participants extended beyond formal research encounters, with the phone serving as a help-line. Over time, this extended to the rest of the research team as it became clear to both study participants and the research assistants that this was an additional avenue for direct representation, enquiry, and advocacy as illustrated below.

'Pork' injections

The routine administration of Heparin following emergency Caesarean section is indicated because of the increased risk of blood clots with potentially fatal complications. As a subgroup, the rates of Caesarean sections are higher in women who are infibulated because of the potential for protracted labour. It is therefore not uncommon for Heparin to be administered to women from the Horn of Africa communities. It came to the attention of a visiting relative (who was a chemist) of an African woman that the preparation of Heparin available at the hospital was porcine based. The patient was extremely distressed to learn about this, refused further treatment and contacted one of the research assistants. It was arranged for a religious leader to visit and reassure the patient that her body was not contaminated and eternally damned as she had not knowingly ingested what was considered *haram* within the Moslem faith. However, the news about the 'pork' injection spread very quickly through her community. In spite of reassurances from religious leaders of the religious dispensation, women were persuaded by others in the community against presenting to the hospital to give birth for fear of an operative birth as well as of the injection (Manderson & Allotey 2003b). One woman stated that she would rather die a good Moslem woman than have her body ritually contaminated and affect her religious standing in the community.

To address this problem, members of the research team convened a meeting with practitioners (medical specialists working with refugee women, pharmacists) and policy advisers to the Department of Health to consider the religious edicts in the assessment of risk of whether a patient needed to be given Heparin, and to explore alternatives to the porcine preparation of Heparin that would be considered acceptable to the community. In the course of the meeting, it was revealed that there were several other medications that were either based on pork products or were immersed in a pork-based medium. The concerns have now been raised with suppliers, who are exploring alternative forms of the medications that can be purchased and this information has been fed back to the women in the community as well as to religious leaders.

The focus of the research on women's reproductive health also enabled the establishment of links with individual women early in pregnancy, and for the links to be sustained with them and other women in the community over time. Accordingly, we met women at community meetings, at informal gatherings and in their homes. By virtue of the subject matter of the research and the relationships that were built, they responded to questions that were often deeply personal, proffering information that was private, painful, problematic, and sometimes provided us with blatant evidence of others' insensitivity or injustice. We followed up on problems wherever appropriate, a situation made possible through links on the advisory committee and a commitment from service providers to work with the research team to find both short and long-term solutions to problems that were identified. This did not always work, as illustrated below.

Zahra's story

Zahra is from the Horn of Africa, and was recruited into the study when she was about seven months pregnant. She had been married for three months in a refugee camp in Sudan, when her husband returned to Eritrea to look after a brother who had been wounded in a 'situation' with the army. She never saw him again and rumour had it that he had been killed. Widowed and alone, she joined the ranks of 'women at risk' (Manderson et al. 1998) and had her application approved to be resettled in Australia. She had not known anyone in Sudan and she knew no one in Australia before her arrival. She met Igor, a Bosnian refugee, early in the settlement process in Australia. Although the level of their spoken English was very basic, they both also spoke some Arabic and managed to communicate sufficiently for Igor to ask and Zahra to accept his marriage proposal.

Eight months after they were married, Zahra became pregnant. With the help of the hospital bicultural worker, she attended regular antenatal clinics and reported a relatively uncomplicated pregnancy. Attendance at the antenatal clinic also presented her with an opportunity to meet other women from similar religious and cultural backgrounds.

In the course of her antenatal care, it was ascertained that she had been infibulated and she was referred to a particular obstetrician. She found the obstetrician very sympathetic; she (the obstetrician) took a Pap smear, which she described as uncomfortable but relatively painless. Through an interpreter, they discussed an option for de-infibulation prior to the birth. Having spoken to the other women in the community, however, she found that this option was discouraged because it was believed to increase the risk of pre-term birth. She therefore decided to wait until she was in labour. The doctor noted this on her patient record as well as her (the doctor's) willingness to be called in when Zahra was due to give birth. When Zahra presented at the onset of labour, she asked through an interpreter if she could be seen by the doctor with whom she was familiar. It was explained to her that since she did not belong to a private insurance fund, she had to be seen by whoever was on duty.

At this point, Zahra telephoned the research assistant working on the project, and asked if she could come in. Igor, she said, was working and would not be given time off to be with her. The research assistant went in to reassure her. The first midwife who started to examine her realised that she was infibulated and explained that she did not feel competent to carry out the examination and would find the resident on duty. The resident attempted a pelvic examination with a speculum in spite of Zahra's screams of pain. The research assistant had to physically restrain him to stop the examination, and asked him to find someone else who knew about infibulation to do the examination. Zahra finally gave birth to a healthy baby girl five hours later, after de-infibulation and an episiotomy. She was then taken to the theatre because of a heavy bleed, probably from retained products of conception. At each stage, the research assistant had to be proactive in enquiring about what was happening in order to explain this to Zahra, although without a clinical background, there was a lot she did not really understand. The research assistant remained with her because the hospital bicultural workers were not available after their scheduled hours. When she eventually had to go home, she made a list of some of the basic needs that Zahra might have and left this with the nurses. Igor was expected to arrive later that evening. Zahra was discharged four days later. Even with the research assistant's support, she had been unable to arrange to see a counsellor or someone with whom she could talk, who could explain to her the implications of de-infibulation and why the birth had been so traumatic.

Zahra was keen to pursue a complaints procedure with some assistance from the research team. While her case has been dealt with to her satisfaction, she wishes to have no more children or any further contact with the health services. She describes the experience as removing most of the joy that giving birth was supposed to bring and she required high levels of emotional and psychological support for at least a year following the birth.

The qualitative design of the study provided us with considerable insight into refugee women's experiences of routine experiences in the labour ward and the points at which possible interventions could be recommended to improve these experiences. The level of involvement also enabled a richer understanding of how reproductive experiences were influenced by their battles with respect also to housing, poverty, unemployment, and loss, grief and loneliness. The longitudinal design of the study with SAME women has enabled contact to be maintained over time, affording the opportunity to follow through cases and to demonstrate good faith through practical returns, and ensuring that women's health concerns were addressed on a case-by-case basis and translated into programs through input into policy debates. Methodologically, the contact also minimised attrition rates in the sample.

Work with refugee and humanitarian immigrant women has an emotional and political intensity. At any given point, on request of the women with whom we were working, we found it necessary to suspend research distance and respond practically. The design of the study was essentially descriptive and was not an intervention study. Indeed the standard requirement for ethics approval requires the institution of mechanisms to deal with untoward effects of the research. However, there are no guidelines for the extension of the role of the researchers to caseworkers. The very reasons for the identification of refugees and humanitarian settlers as an important population for research (that is, their vulnerability, marginalisation and consequently poor access to services) provide the rationale for the need to review ethical obligations of researchers in working with them. While it is possible to present participants with a list of possible points of referral, there is a need to re-evaluate the level of involvement of researchers in facilitating that process.

Cross-cultural research and marginalised populations

While qualitative methodology attempts to address the power relations in research through the establishment of rapport between the researchers and participants, the shifting of the balance of power can also raise questions of dependency. Due to the level of trust, for instance, some of the women thought they did not need to sign consent forms for participation because we would not be asking them to participate in a project that would not benefit or indeed harm them. Similar trust was placed in researchers when HIV positive pregnant women in Ivory Coast provided 'informed consent' to participate in a placebo controlled trial for vertical transmission. In interviews following the cessation of the trial, women reported that they did not believe that foreign researchers would provide them with a drug (placebo) that was not effective, knowing that they were HIV positive, needed treatment and would not want the virus to be transmitted to their unborn infants (French 1997; Lurie & Wolfe 1997).

Other issues highlighted have been addressed in research with indigenous Australians, developed in the context of community criticism of the conventional conduct of medical research. In the past, substantial research has been undertaken with Aborigines and Torres Strait Islanders, but with little consultation with communities about their own perceived needs, without community involvement in the conceptualisation or design of research, and with no direct impact on health policies or programs. Indigenous Australians questioned the ethical practices of researchers, and sought and gained Federal Government agreement that in future, research practice should honour the principles of community determination, ensure community involvement in the formulation of research and the collection of data (both biomedical and social), and ensure feedback and benefits to the community. These agreements were incorporated into a number of important policy documents and the procedural guidelines of the peak National Health and Medical Research Council (NHMRC 1991; Rowse 1992).

While the importance of uniform guidelines is not in question, working cross-culturally does raise unique issues that need to be acknowledged also by tertiary institutions and funding agencies. Current research funding precludes the possibility of intervention unless the research design is specifically an intervention study. Funding that would cover any casework performed by the research team, for instance, cannot be built into grant applications. Similarly, any advantages to the community that result from the research are not considered outcomes of research at the institutional level, which values mainly academic research publications and continued competitive grant funding often at the expense of 'giving back to the community'.

Conclusions

The outcomes of the research were to enable data collected to assist in the determination of predictors of well-being in the short and longer term, and to identify problems that continue to affect women's reproductive health in the course of their settlement into Australian society. As we have described, information necessarily needed to be fed to service providers regularly through the course of the project, because of the urgency of individuals who had come to us for assistance and because of the community's expectations. The emotional density of field research with vulnerable populations needs a methodological shift. The researcher is absolutely dependent on the community with whom she or he works, if only to accept their presence and provide them with information.

Research with this community should be designed to enable an improvement of social links given previously identified problems of social isolation (Allotey 1998). Minimally, the research should allow the inclusion of at least one extra person into the participant's social network, one who could assist in negotiating barriers to access.

Global trends in the number of refugees and asylum seekers combined with geopolitical forces and human rights discourses have made refugee health one of the fastest growing areas of public health practice and research. With this growth come some major challenges that require innovation and lateral thinking in all areas, including standard guidelines for ethical research. In countries such as Australia that have strict regulations for the treatment of onshore asylum seekers, there is the potential for ethical dilemmas to arise between researchers' perceived ethical or humanitarian obligations to research communities and contradicting policies. These issues need careful consideration in the planning and implementation of research projects.

Acknowledgments

The authors would like to acknowledge the invaluable assistance of Samia Baho and Lourice Demian in conducting the research and liaising with women in the various communities.

Recommended reading

Manderson, L,. Kirk, M. & Hoban, E. (2001) Walking the Talk: Research partnerships in women's business, In Dyck, I., Lewis, N.D. & McLafferty, S. (eds) *Geographies of Women's Health* Routledge, New York and London, pp. 177–94.

Manderson, L. & Wilson, R. (1998) Negotiating with Communities: The politics and ethics of research, *Human Organization*, 57(2): 215.

UNHCR (1999) New Issues in Refugee Research: Working Paper no 1 Centre for Documentation and Research, UNHCR, Geneva.

World Health Organisation (1999) Putting Women First: Ethical and Safety Recommendations for Research on Domestic Violence Against Women, World Health Organisation, Geneva, pp. 1-13.

References

ABS (1996) Basic community profile series, Australian Bureau of Statistics, Canberra.

Allotey, P. (1998) Travelling with excess baggage: a study of refugee women in Western Australia, *Women and Health*, 28(2): 63–81.

Australia NHMRC (National Health and Medical Research Committee) (1991) Guidelines on ethical matters in Aboriginal and Torres Strait Islander Health Research, Approved by the 111th Session of the National Health and Medical Research Council, Brisbane, June AGPS, Canberra.

Corkery, E., Palmer, C., Foley, M.E., Schechter, C.B., Frisher, L. & Roman, S.H. (1997) Effect of bicultural community health worker on completion of diabetes education in a hispanic population, *Diabetes Care*, 20(3): 254–7.

French, H. (1997) AIDS research in Africa: Juggling risks and hopes, In *New York Times*, p. 1.

Kelaher, M. & Manderson, L. (2000) Migration and mainstreaming: matching health services to immigrants' needs in Australia, *Health Policy*, 54: 1–11.

Lurie, P. & Wolfe, S. (1997) Unethical trials of interventions to reduce perinatal transmission of the human immunodeficiency virus in developing countries, *New England Journal of Medicine,* 337: 853–5.

Manderson, L. & Allotey, P. (2003a) The cultural politics of competence in Australian health services, *Anthropology in Medicine*, 10(1): 70–85.

Manderson, L. & Allotey, P. (2003b) Story telling, marginality and community in Australia: how immigrants position their differences in health care settings, *Medical Anthropology*, 22: 1–21.

Manderson, L., Kelaher, M., Markovic, M. & McManus, K. (1998) A Woman without a Man is a Woman at Risk: Women at Risk in Australian Humanitarian Programs, *Journal of Refugee Studies*, 11(3): 267–83.

Manderson, L., Kirk, M. & Hoban, E. (2001) Walking the Talk: Research partnerships in women's business, In Dyck, I., Lewis, N.D. & McLafferty, S. (eds) *Geographies of Women's Health*, Routledge, New York and London, pp. 177–94.

Manderson, L. & Wilson, R. (1998) Negotiating with Communities: The politics and ethics of research, *Human Organization*, 57(2): 215.

Musser-Granski, J. & Carillo, D.F. (1997) The use of bilingual, bicultural paraprofessionals in mental health services: issues for hiring, training and supervision, *Community Mental Health Journal*, 33(1): 51–60.

Riddick, S. (1998) Improving access for limited English-speaking consumers: a review of strategies in health care settings, *Journal of Health Care for the Poor and Underserved*, 9(Supplement): S40-S61.

Roberts, H. (ed) (1981) *Doing feminist research*, Routledge & Kegan Paul, London and Boston.

Rowse, T. (1992) The Royal Commission, ATSIC and self-determination: A review of the Royal Commission into Aboriginal deaths in custody, *Australian Journal of Social Issues*, 27(3): 153–72.

Tribe, R. (1999) Bridging the gap or damming the flow? Some observations on using interpreters/bicultural workers when working with refugee clients, many of whom have been tortured, *British Journal of Medical Psychology*, 72: 567–76.

14

Controlling Compassion: the Media, Refugees, and Asylum Seekers

Peter Mares and Pascale Allotey

By its very nature, the mass displacement of human populations destroys the normal and largely predictable patterns of daily existence. The effect on those immediately involved has been largely the subject of this text. For those not directly affected by such processes, the experience is usually communicated via the media. Since television brought the Vietnam War into Western lounge rooms, audiences have been witness to ever more confronting and vivid images of armed conflict, ethnic and communal violence, man-made catastrophes and natural disasters. With the advent of international satellite television networks like CNN, which also provide footage to domestic television networks worldwide, and with the technological revolution in real time communications, images and descriptions of human suffering and vulnerability reach global audiences in ever increasing volume and with ever greater immediacy. Public reaction to this kind of 'front-line' reporting is highly variable and depends on presentation, interpretation, and the external political climate (Kleinman & Kleinman 1997). The contradictions are manifest in our everyday experience. In some cases, such as during the Live Aid concerts organised by Sir Bob Geldof, images of starving children have motivated millions to dig deep and donate record amounts of money to charity. At other times, similar images of large numbers of displaced people, including children, have not only failed to engender any great show of public sympathy and hospitality, but have instead inspired antipathy and fear. Audiences may be transfixed by the drama of a solo adventurer awaiting rescue mid ocean in the capsized hull of a state-of-the art yacht, yet pictures of asylum seekers chancing their lives in unseaworthy vessels on the high seas are more likely to prompt demands for tougher measures to deter illegal immigrants than pressure to lift quotas for the resettlement of refugees. These examples demonstrate the power of the media to shape attitudes and opinions in apparently unpredictable and often contradictory ways. While the media often claims to be in the business of conveying objective 'news' and 'information', this public interest role often stands in conflict with the desire to engage and hold audiences. The use of emotionally charged imagery and gripping narrative technique gives the media capacity to enlighten and to mislead in equal measure. In more subtle ways it gives the media the power to shape public debate on humanitarian obligations and so exert a profound influence on policy outcomes (O'Shaughnessy 1999).

Humanitarian obligations can only be met by the identification of vulnerable populations and the development of policy that allows intervention. In the public health arena, as in other sectors, policy development should be a process designed to guide decision making based on the best available evidence. At best, it is based on balanced and accurate information, but remains dynamic and responsive to changing contexts. At its worst, it is ad hoc, hostage to vested interests or political agendas and influenced by insufficient or misinterpreted information (Gardner 1997). In reality, politics plays a major role in policy development and the media therefore has a significant influence on the outcomes. It can help to ensure that policy is relevant by giving voice to community concerns, or it can distort policy by exaggerating and inflaming community sentiment. The media has the capacity to act as a disinterested player, stimulating productive public debate, but is vulnerable to influence and manipulation by powerful actors, including government. This is nowhere more evident than in the development of policy towards refugees and asylum seekers.

Taking examples of reporting on refugee issues, including specific health related news items, this chapter describes the role of the media in shaping public perception of refugees and asylum seekers. From a public health perspective, this is important because an essential element of public health is advocacy for vulnerable groups to ensure equity in the allocation of health resources to address their needs (Beaglehole & Bonita 1997). The perceptions of the broader community, not directly affected by refugee crises, influences the extent to which humanitarian obligations are met both within the context of a humanitarian emergency and in the resettlement of displaced persons. Specific instances are highlighted and discussed. The chapter also discusses the roles of different actors such as humanitarian agencies, advocacy groups, and politicians and their use of the media in recent debates about refugees and asylum seekers. The available evidence on the effect of the media on the health of refugees and asylum seekers is presented and some strategies proposed for public health advocacy groups who wish to promote more constructive media coverage.

A khaki election

On 10 November 2001 Australians voted in an extraordinary federal election. Rather than the traditional focus on domestic issues like taxation levels or spending on health and education, the campaign was largely fought on issues of national security and border protection. The international backdrop to the campaign was the US-led military offensive in Afghanistan (for which Australia volunteered troops) following the September 11 terror attacks in New York and Washington. The domestic context was an atmosphere of panic about the unauthorised arrival of mostly Middle Eastern asylum seekers on Australian territory at the rate of a few hundred people per month.[1] Within 48 hours of the September 11 attacks, Australia's Defence Minister Peter Reith had drawn an explicit link between the two, warning that the unauthorised arrival of boats on Australian territory 'can be a pipeline for terrorists to come in and use your country as a staging post for terrorist activities'.[2] The irony that Afghan asylum seekers were fleeing the very same 'terror' regime that Australia was helping to fight did not appear to concern him.

Neither did it worry Australia's 'shock-jocks', the prime-time millionaire talkback hosts who dominate the airwaves on commercial radio. On 12 September Alan Jones, the top-rating breakfast host on Sydney radio, confidently declared that the terror attacks had been carried out by 'sleepers', terrorists who had been living quietly in the United States for years. Turning to the Australian context, he then posed the following rhetorical question: 'How many of these Afghan boat people are "sleepers"?'[3] Prime Minister John Howard revived the theme just a few days before polling day, telling Brisbane's *Courier Mail* newspaper that '[y]ou don't know who is coming [on the boats] and you don't know whether they do have terrorist links or not…'[4]

The campaign for Australia's 10 November federal election also followed in the wake of the *Tampa* affair, when the Australian Government used the navy to prevent a Norwegian container ship, the MV *Tampa*, from landing 433 asylum seekers at the Australian Indian Ocean territory of Christmas Island. On 26 August 2001 the *Tampa* rescued the asylum seekers from their sinking wooden ferry after being alerted to their plight by the Australian search and rescue organisation. However, the Australian Government insisted that the *Tampa* return the asylum seekers to a port in Indonesia, rather than bring them to the closer port of Christmas Island. After a standoff lasting three days, the ship's master defied the Australian authorities and steamed towards Christmas Island, arguing that his rescued passengers required urgent medical treatment. The Australian Government responded by sending elite SAS troops to board his vessel.

The *Tampa* affair marked a fundamental turning point in Australia's refugee policy. The Prime Minister John Howard declared that asylum seekers rescued by the *Tampa* would not set foot on the Australian mainland, and instead naval vessels were used to transport them to Nauru and New Zealand. Australia then adopted the same approach to all subsequent vessels attempting to carry asylum seekers to its territory from Indonesia. The vessels were boarded by Australian naval personnel and told that they must return to Indonesia. In some cases warning shots were fired over the bows. If boats persisted in entering Australia's 12-mile exclusion zone, then they were boarded at sea and forcibly turned around. If the Australian Navy was unable to convince or force the boats back to Indonesia, or if the boats foundered, then the asylum seekers were transferred to navy ships and taken to detention centres in Nauru, or subsequently, Papua New Guinea (Mares 2001).

Amid the fears and uncertainties unleashed by the September 11 terror attacks, the tough line on 'boat people' proved enormously popular with voters. As the *Australian* newspaper commented, it represented 'one of the Government's chief claims to national leadership' and was the 'main preoccupation' of the election campaign.[5] The government used the rhetoric of 'border security' at every available opportunity, often demonising vulnerable people in the process. For example, on 7 October 2001, in the first days of the election campaign, the Minister for Immigration Philip Ruddock announced that a group of asylum seekers trying to reach Australia had thrown children overboard 'in a clearly planned and premeditated' attempt to force their way into Australia.[6] The story made immediate headlines and two days later, on 9 October, Prime Minister John Howard declared on radio 'I certainly don't want people of that type in Australia, I really don't'. On 10 October Defence Minister Peter Reith released photographs of children in the sea wearing life jackets, which he presented as documentary proof of what had happened. He told ABC radio 774 in Melbourne that '[w]e have a number of people, obviously RAN [Royal Australian Navy] people, who were there who reported the children were thrown into the water'. Yet serious doubts had emerged about the veracity of the original reports immediately after they were made public, and in fact, the 'evidence' on which the immigration minister, the defence minister and the prime minister had based their initial public statements was third hand conversations, the veracity of which they made no attempt to check. After the election, it was revealed that the photographic 'evidence' of children in the water was from a separate incident, the following day, when the children were rescued after their boat sank. Military officers and senior public servants were aware that the reports of children being thrown overboard were untrue and that the photographs did not depict such an event. To varying degrees they had tried to correct the public 'mistake' of their political masters before the election. However, the three relevant ministers—the prime minister and the ministers for Defence and Immigration—claim this advice never reached them. By the time the story was corrected, the election was over and the government had been returned to office. No apology was made to the asylum seekers for the way in which they had been so publicly wronged.

The *Tampa* affair and its aftermath provide a particularly blatant example of the way in which the plight of vulnerable people can be exploited to serve a political agenda—in this case the re-election of a conservative coalition government. However, the effects of such a strategy last well beyond polling day. The deliberate polarisation of opinion serves to constrain constructive debate on the policy challenges posed by refugees and asylum seekers who arrive in the country without authorisation. Any hint of compassion towards displaced people is construed as weakness on the issue of border security, limiting the opportunities for reasoned discussion of alternative approaches to a complex humanitarian problem, and even reducing tolerance for the expression of different viewpoints. Almost one full year after the *Tampa* affair, a suburban library in Canberra was forced to dismantle a public display sympathetic to the plight of asylum seekers held in Australia's immigration detention centres. Some members of the public were so incensed by the display that they subjected library staff to verbal abuse and threats of violence.[7]

Sections of the media offered vociferous support to the Australian Government in its hardline response to the *Tampa*; other media outlets were decidedly critical of its approach. Either way, the welfare of the 433 asylum seekers rescued at sea became subsidiary to the drama being played in the waters off Christmas Island. Meanwhile, anecdotal evidence suggests that some refugees already living in Australia were deeply distressed by the unfolding saga and the often acrimonious debate it aroused in the Australian community. One Syrian refugee, who had himself originally arrived in Australia by boat 18 months earlier, says the *Tampa* affair made him feel insecure and unwelcome in Australia. It reawakened traumatic experiences of his own flight to safety and caused him such emotional upheaval that he was compelled to ask his doctor to prescribe him sleeping tablets in order to get to sleep at night.[8]

Pariahs, parasites, or pitiable

The demonisation of refugees and asylum seekers for political gain may have reached its apotheosis during Australia's 2001 federal election campaign, but the practice was already firmly entrenched. The media has often been complicit in this process.

There are numerous examples of well-researched reporting on the asylum seeker issue. Many journalists have made persistent efforts to expose the problems in Australia's immigration detention centres and to give voice to the asylum seekers themselves. They have raised questions about the cost and efficacy of Australia's harsh policy of mandatory detention for all non-citizens who arrive in the country without valid travel documents, including those who seek protection under the provisions of the 1951 Geneva Convention on Refugees[9] (UNHCR 1951). Many journalists are affronted at government attempts to manipulate coverage of the issue, for example, by banning media access to the detention centres, or by attempting to prevent any photographs from being taken that might 'humanise or personalise' asylum seekers.[10] In the face of these clumsy attempts at media control, many journalists and editors have done their best to promote sober and rational debate about what is a complex humanitarian issue—how to deal with the unauthorised movement of people across Australia's borders. However, the media has also been responsible for peddling myths and exaggerating fears.

'Typhoid found in refugee centres' (McKinnon 2001) was the title of an exclusive story describing the high prevalence of infectious diseases over an eighteen-month period in a population of asylum seekers in immigration detention. The diseases included typhoid, tuberculosis, and hepatitis B and C. The story appeared in Brisbane's *Courier Mail* newspaper, warning of the exotic and deadly diseases carried by immigration detainees awaiting determination of their appeals to seek asylum in Australia under the Refugee Convention.

The story highlights a number of issues. In reality, of the 'almost 1000 cases' reported in the article, there were ten cases of typhoid and eight of active tuberculosis. Most of the other cases posed minimal public health risk, a detail not clarified by the story. The central message of the story was to convey the potential threat of the asylum seekers to Australian society. This message was further reinforced by comments from politicians on the importance of isolating these people to protect the wider community.

Secondly, the confusion created by the interchangeable and indiscriminate use of the terms 'refugees', 'asylum seekers' and 'illegal immigrants' has been widely documented in many developed countries as an important factor fuelling the rise of the conservative right and associated anti-immigration sentiment (de Bousingen 2002; Mares 2001; McMaster 2001; Steiner 2000). In Australia the use of the term 'queue jumper' has been particularly powerful, cultivating an image of outsiders who refuse to obey the common rules of courtesy critical to social membership and who thus should remain excluded. The at times deliberate blurring of terminology results in a uniform labelling of distrust and illegitimacy, and creates an ideal attribute for prejudice and stigmatisation.

In contrast, a story about the discovery of infectious diseases in a 'refugee centre' *could* invoke the sympathy of the audience, and may involve an implied or explicit call for humanitarian intervention. This is more likely in a context where the subject of the report is far removed from its audience; where the news story deals with a refugee health crisis safely contained in a distant land. It is almost as if there is an inverse relationship between the degree of compassion shown for the plight of displaced people and the proximity with which their plight is viewed. The closer they are, the more likely it is that sympathy will be displaced by antipathy. The media, and media audiences, are comfortable with images of refugees and asylum seekers as helpless and bedraggled. Politicians contrast the 'queue jumper' on our shores with the stereotype image of refugees 'waiting patiently' in squalid refugee camps far away. These deserving refugees are portrayed as passive. We can choose to bestow our generosity upon them or we can choose to withhold it. In other words they are—or at least they appear to be—subject to our control. By contrast those who take the initiative, arriving uninvited and 'unprocessed' on Australia's shores display a disagreeable degree of self-will. The willingness of some refugees to take action to address their situation breaks the comfortable stereotype of passivity in which the media and its audience usually seek to contain them.

Benevolence or malevolence?

It is illuminating here to draw a comparison between the generous public response to the so-called 'safe haven' refugees brought to Australia from Kosovo and East Timor in 1999[11] and the animosity shown to 'boat people' from Afghanistan, Iraq and Iran who arrived 'uninvited' at around the same time. The safe haven refugees were landed in Australia as part of a government sponsored relief effort. They were allowed entry into the country on specially created safe haven visas which prevented them from applying to reside in the country on any other grounds, including as refugees under the convention (Mares 2001, Head 1999). The fate of the safe haven refugees rested almost entirely in the hands of the minister for immigration who could shorten, extend, or cancel their entry visas without any recourse to the courts. They were housed in disused military barracks, generally at some distance from major cities. These safe haven refugees were thus largely confined to the role of passive and grateful recipients of Australian largesse, and so held within the bounds of the dominant media stereotype of refugees described above. When some of the temporary evacuees did complain about their treatment, this was portrayed as a demonstration of ingratitude.

By contrast, boat people from the Middle East landed in Australia in an unregulated and apparently uncontrollable manner. The media frequently resorted to metaphors of natural disaster and war to record their arrival. There was talk of a 'flood tide' of boat people, who threatened to 'inundate' Australia in 'waves' (Mares 2001 p. 27). Government responses to refugees and asylum seekers are based not only on the magnitude of the crisis and humanitarianism, but also on the internal economic interests and political agenda of the potential host country (Shacknove 1993) and in the two cases under discussion, it is apparent that media reporting and public perceptions were also influenced by official attitudes. The minister for immigration described the arrival of the boat people as 'a national emergency' and an 'assault on our borders', while the first safe haven refugees were personally welcomed to Australia by the prime minister.

At another level, detailed and very immediate reporting of the Kosovo and East Timor conflicts had given Australians a narrative structure in which to place the safe haven refugees as innocent victims of aggression. By comparison, when it was reported at all, the tragedy of Afghanistan was portrayed as a long-running saga with no obvious beginning or end point. The country was generally presented as a site of intractable conflict, in which individual actors could not easily be identified or ascribed with motives. As a legacy of the Gulf War, sympathy for people suffering under the regime of Saddam Hussein was tempered by the identification of the country as a whole as an aggressor and an enemy.

Australia was not the only developed nation where Kosovo refugees were 'popular' while refugees from elsewhere remained 'unpopular'. Gibney (1999) describes how 'the river of hostility' towards asylum seekers and refugees in Europe suddenly 'started to flow backwards' when refugees began to flee Kosovo in large numbers in March 1999. He identifies official attitudes as central to this change of public mood, as European governments replaced the rhetoric of border control and exclusion with practical action to assist in a humanitarian crisis. Gibney identifies a number of reasons for this. The first is 'regionality'. The proximity of the Kosovo crisis required countries in Western Europe to develop a more organised and coherent response to the refugee outflow from Kosovo, rather than risk the spontaneous, large-scale movement of refugees spilling across the continent. In other words, it was in the political and economic interests of host governments to convince their citizens that the Kosovars should be welcomed. Secondly, Gibney notes that European governments were 'implicated' in the Kosovo tragedy, because the NATO bombing campaign turned the threat of mass expulsion of Kosovars 'into an immediate and pressing reality'. As NATO had used the language of 'humanitarian values' to intervene in Kosovo in the first place, it was thus 'hard for Western states to deny a duty to ease the plight of the displaced' (Gibney 1999). Finally Gibney identifies the issue of 'relatedness' (which others have more bluntly described as 'race'), arguing that the response to the Kosovars was sympathetic because they were seen as fellow Europeans: 'people sharing a common civilization and culture'. While African refugees remain 'alien' and 'enigmatic' to European audiences, here were 'forced migrants who looked and dressed like them ... and who, through the use of articulate and well-educated translators, could express their suffering in terms that resonated with Western audiences' (Gibney 1999).

Media and policy

In the examples above we have examined the interaction between official attitudes, media imagery and public perception, describing the ways in which political leadership can set the tone for news reports, and how this in turn can shape the popular response to a particular instance of human displacement and suffering. This suggests that the relationship between policy formation and media coverage is by no means simple or linear as suggested by terms such as 'the CNN effect'.

Arnot argues that 'the television camera has become the single most powerful weapon many of the world's refugees will ever encounter'. The 'miracle of live TV' can bind 'viewer and victim ... together in time and space', so that Americans see children dying as they eat their breakfast and are propelled into action. Arnot believes that if television networks would devote more energy and resources to covering stories of famine and conflict, then the Western world would exhibit a swifter and more compassionate response to humanitarian emergencies (Arnot 1995). However, detailed investigation suggests that the relationship between reporting, public compassion, and government response is not nearly so straightforward.

One of the most celebrated examples of the alleged power of the 'CNN effect' was the US intervention in Somalia 1992, and the ignominious withdrawal of US forces some months later. According to Arnot, the marines arrived 'after a veritable media blitz' of images of starving children denied food by armed warlords, but were soon forced to retreat again because, in 'the most horrendous example of "pack" journalism', the media drew the simple conclusion US forces 'don't belong in Somalia' (Arnot 1995). However, Mermin shows that the interest of US television networks in Somalia was in fact preceded by expressions of concern about the situation in the country which were voiced by influential actors in Washington.

'[T]he evidence indicates that before television made the decision to cover the crisis in Somalia, influential politicians had spoken out on it, indicating to journalists who routinely look to Washington for possible stories that Somalia constituted a significant concern of American foreign policy and that it warranted consideration for space in the news...' (Mermin 1997).

In other words, the media was not simply responding to an extreme case of human suffering in Somalia. Editorial decisions to focus on events there were influenced by the prior concern of powerful players in Washington who wanted to move Somalia higher up the foreign policy agenda of the US Government. Neuman points out that if television reporting forced President George Bush (senior) to intervene in Somalia, then there should have been a similar response to the equally horrific and equally prolific television images of starving families in Sudan, but there was not (Neuman 1996). She argues that the frequent refrain: 'Pictures got us in [to Somalia], pictures got us out' does not accord with a 'more textured' reality and the sudden US withdrawal from Somalia (under President Bill Clinton) was not the inevitable result of television footage 'of an American soldier's corpse being dragged through the streets of Mogadishu' as is often claimed. Neuman maintains that Clinton could have used the influence of his office to counter the power of that image, but chose instead to *allow* the pictures to dominate, not wishing to 'expend his political capital' on an issue that was 'the legacy of an earlier administration' (Neuman 1996).

Mermin and Neuman do not deny that the media exerts an influence on policy formation, nor do they present journalists as simple tools in the hands of politicians. Rather, they argue that the interaction between media and government is far more complex. Editorial decisions are not insulated from the politics, and nor is it inevitable that politicians will succumb to the power of media images.

Robinson suggests that exaggeration of the 'CNN effect' is significant for humanitarians who 'seek to harness the perceived potential of the news media to facilitate humanitarian action' (Robinson 2000). If the sheer volume and power of media images of human suffering are no guarantee of government action, how can the relationship between media reporting and government decision making be better understood? In order to answer this question, Robinson attempts to identify the conditions under which the media can have a decisive impact on policy. Under his model, media influence is greatest in situations where a government's policy line is 'uncertain' and where 'news reports are critically framed, advocating a particular course of action'. By contrast, media influence is likely to be minimal in situations where the executive has already decided on a particular course of action: 'When the government has clear and well-articulated objectives it tends to set the news agenda' (Robinson 2000). In other words, if there is a lack of consensus over policy within the elite ranks of decision makers, then there is a much greater prospect of media influence:

> By promoting a particular policy line advocated either by elites outside the executive or particular members of the executive itself, the media can play a key role in causing policy change.
>
> (Robinson 2000)

Robinson's model fits with events surrounding the Australian Government's decision to offer temporary safe haven to refugees from Kosovo in 1999. Australia had not previously confronted the difficult questions posed by the Kosovo crisis, of whether to provide short-term sanctuary to those fleeing an immediate crisis, and the government was slow to take decisive action. As viewers watched the distressing television footage of refugees streaming out of Kosovo, the media portrayed the government as mean and hard-hearted and radio talkback lines ran hot with criticism. The effect of media reporting reached into the lounge rooms of the elite. As politicians returned home to celebrate Easter with their families, they faced questions from their children about why Australia was doing so little to help (Shanahan 1999). A cabinet meeting on the first working day after Easter decided to offer a temporary safe haven for 4000 Kosovar refugees. Whether this media driven response was the best policy outcome remains a matter of debate.

In contrast, the limits on the media's power to determine policy were evident when it was time for the safe haven refugees to be sent home. The media was generally very critical of the government's decision to return the Kosovars, arguing that it was too early to do so. However, on this occasion there was no uncertainty in government policy (and so a necessary condition for media influence under Robinson's model was absent). The government was resolute in its decision to remove the Kosovars from Australia and carried it through, although media and public criticism did achieve concessions for a small number of people suffering serious illnesses or displaying severe psychological problems arising from their experiences of trauma (Mares 2001 p. 162).

Policy, rights, and public health

The policies developed to guide decisions about the extent of the generosity of the receiving government and community have obvious effects on health and well-being. They determine the level of access to public goods including health care and related services such as housing, education, and welfare services and they control the level of enjoyment of human rights taken for granted by citizens. They also make an explicit statement of the value of different groups within a community. Non-citizens are seen as competitors for scarce public goods. As Thomas (2001) writes, displaced people:

> ...are not an acknowledged part of any society, and therefore, cannot claim even the basic right to life itself because they are not citizens of a legitimate, 'nation'. Furthermore, their position is weakened by the sometimes 'real' sometimes 'imagined' impact that their presence has on the livelihood of 'legitimate' nationals inhabiting those areas close to a refugee camp.
>
> (Thomas 2001)

As people without entitlement, refugee non-citizens are only acceptable in a certain guise—as the passive and grateful recipients of the generosity—which we, as citizens, might choose to bestow. Given that a relatively high proportion of asylum seekers who make it to Australia on their own have legitimate claims to asylum, the receptiveness of the host community is important regardless of the visa status of an individual at a given point in time. If made to feel unwelcome, notions of trust, reciprocity and engagement with the broader community, shattered prior to seeking asylum, are more difficult to rebuild. The flow-on effects include marginalised communities unable or reluctant to participate in the wider society; a phenomenon that has already been documented in the growing body of literature on the effects of social inequalities on health that also begin to explore the concepts of social capital, social cohesion and how they influence health and well-being (Allotey 2003; Berkman & Kawachi 2000; Harris & Telfer 2001; Mateen & Titemore 1999).

While there has been extensive documentation on the poor health and barriers to accessing health and health related facilities for minority groups, what is less well documented is the effect on the marginalisation of minorities on the dominant group. Based on an analysis of data from several states in the US, Reidpath (2003) reports that mortality in dominant groups is higher where there are larger numbers of disenfranchised groups and postulates that policies of exclusion have flow-on effects not only on the minority group but also ultimately on the whole population

(Reidpath 2003). Policies implemented now in response to the current refugee crisis can therefore be expected to have longer-term implications on the broader society.

Conclusion: the limits of influence and the responsibility of public health advocates

From the above discussion it becomes apparent that media reporting can shape public perceptions of refugees and asylum seekers. On the one hand, compassionate and sympathetic coverage can help to promote understanding and encourage generous assistance to refugees and others in need, resulting in public pressure for the increased protection *of* refugees. One the other hand, the portrayal of displaced people as a potential threat, and as competitors for scarce public goods, can generate and intensify feelings of fear, and awaken popular demands for protection *from* refugees. Yet while the media can influence public policy on refugee issues, it has no overwhelming power to do so. Its influence is likely to be greatest where policy differences already exist within the ranks of executive government and other members of the decision making elite. Conversely, political leaders often enjoy success in seeking to influence media coverage in ways sympathetic to their own political agenda.

What lessons can be drawn from this for public health advocates wishing to use the media to influence government action? Firstly, it should be recognised that while journalists are often accused of 'hunting in packs', and media ownership is increasingly concentrated in fewer hands, there remains a degree of diversity within the media landscape as was evident in media coverage of the *Tampa* affair.

Secondly, it must be recognised that most media outlets are driven by the commercial imperative to maximise its audience or readership and so win advertising dollars. Even public sector broadcasters (such as the ABC and BBC) must justify their tax-payer funds with evidence that they are winning a significant share of the available audience. The media is in the business of maintaining market share by making news coverage entertaining as well as informative and most media work under intense and ever intensifying time pressures. This encourages sensationalism, simplification, stereotyping, and an over-reliance on 'official sources' in place of time consuming investigative reporting.

Thirdly, it must be recognised that media's power to shape policy is often exaggerated and that politicians shape the media agenda in significant ways. One way of working with these day-to-day realities is to train humanitarian workers in media skills, to increase their chances of delivering the message that they set out to convey, rather than feed into a dominant news agenda or a pre-conceived notion of what the story is about (Phillips 2000). This helps to impart an understanding of such issues as the constraints imposed by tight deadlines, the editorial pressure to find a fresh angle on a story, the need for attributed quotes, and the voracious appetite for engaging or dramatic pictures. If those who advocate on behalf of vulnerable people also understand the way in which the media works then they may be in a position to exert greater influence over what finally gets published or broadcast (Chapman & Lupton 1994). A complementary approach is to seek meetings with senior editors in an attempt to influence the overall shape and direction of editorial policy.

It is almost a default setting for the media to cast events in binary terms—'good' versus 'bad', 'victims' versus 'perpetrators', 'innocent' versus 'guilty'. This creates an engaging narrative framework in which to develop a story, but does little to convey the complexity of humanitarian emergencies or to foster rational debate on appropriate policy responses. Ferris argues that this approach is often encouraged by humanitarian agencies themselves, albeit with the best of intentions:

> It's very effective…in fund-raising to show images of children, who are suffering, who are hungry, with the unspoken and often spoken message that by contributing money you can ease the situation of this child.[12]

When humanitarian agencies take journalists to sites of human suffering, they often do so with the aim of encouraging donations for relief efforts. Equally, they run the risk that a report on a situation of despair and desperation can engender 'compassion fatigue'. Alternatively, it might bring a sudden rush of charitable donations, yet confirm stereotypes of refugees as passive innocents. The flip side of this stereotype is the menacing image of the queue jumper. As long as the romantic notion of refugees in distant lands as 'smiling and very grateful and quiet'[13] persists, then audiences in the developed world will continue to be disconcerted by the real refugees who make it to their shores.

Recommended reading

Chapman, S. & Lupton, D. (1994) *The fight for public health. Principles and practice of media advocacy*, BMJ Publishing Group, London.

Jupp, J. (2002) *From White Australia to Woomera: the story of Australian immigration*, Cambridge University Press, Melbourne.

Mares, P. (2002) *Borderline*, UNSW Press, Sydney.

McMaster, D. (2001) *Asylum seekers. Australia's response to refugees*, Melbourne University Press, Melbourne.

References

Allotey, P. (2003) Refugee health, In Teadtke, J.A. (ed), *Encyclopedia of Medical Anthropology*, Kluwer, New Haven CT.

Arnot, B. (1995) *Waiting for the Cameras: Journalism and Humanitarian Crises. World Refugee Survey 1995*, US Committee for Refugees, Washington DC.

Beaglehole, R. & Bonita, R. (1997) *Public Health at the Crossroads. Achievements and Prospects*, Cambridge University Press, Cambridge.

Berkman, L. & Kawachi, I. (eds.) (2000) *Social Epidemiology*, Oxford University Press, New York.

Chapman, S. & Lupton, D. (1994) *The fight for public health. Principles and practice of media advocacy*, BMJ Publishing Group, London.

de Bousingen, D.D. (2002) Health issues and the rise of Le Pen in France, *Lancet*, 359: 1673.

Gardner, H. (1997) Introduction, In Gardner, H. (ed) *Health Policy in Australia*, Oxford University Press, Melbourne, pp. 1–10.

Gibney, M.J. (1999) Kosovo and beyond: popular and unpopular refugees, *Forced Migration Review*, 5(August): 28–31.

Harris, M.F. & Telfer, B.L. (2001) The health of asylum seekers living in the community, *Medical Journal of Australia*, 175: 589–92.

Kleinman, A. & Kleinman, J. (1997) The appeal of experience: the dismay of images: cultural appropriations of suffering in our times, In Kleinman, A., Das, V. & Lock, M. (eds), *Social Suffering*, University of California Press, Berkeley, pp. 1–23.

Mares, P. (2001) *Borderline*, UNSW Press, Sydney.

Mateen, F. & Titemore, B .(1999) The right to seek asylum: a dwindling right? *Brief, Centre for Human Rights and Humanitarian Law*, 2: 2.

McKinnon, M. (2001) Typhoid found in refugee centres, In the *Courier Mail* Brisbane, 23 June.

McMaster, D. (2001) *Asylum seekers. Australia's response to refugees*, Melbourne University Press, Melbourne.

Mermin, J. (1997) Television News and American Intervention in Somalia: The Myth of a Media-Driven Foreign Policy, *Political Science Quarterly*, 112(3): 385–403.

Neuman, J. (1996) *Lights, Camera, War: Is Media Technology Driving International Politics?*, St Martin's Press, New York.

O'Shaughnessy, M. (1999) Defining the media, In *Media and Society*, Oxford University Press, Melbourne, pp. 2–30.

Phillips, M. (2000) Working with the media: notes for refugee advocates, *Forced Migration Review*, 8 (December): 33–4.

Reidpath, D. (2003) (forthcoming) Love thy neighbour, it's good for your health, *Social Science & Medicine*.

Robinson, P. (2000) The Policy-Media Interaction Model: Measuring Media Power During Humanitarian Crisis, *Journal of Peace Research*, 37(5): 613–33.

Shacknove, A. (1993) From asylum to containment, *International Journal of Refugee Law*, 5(4): 516–33.

Shanahan, D. (1999) Anyone who had a heart, In the *Australian*, Sydney, 10 April.

Steiner, N. (2000) *Arguing about asylum: the complexity of refugee debates in Europe*, St Martin's Press, New York.

Thomas, P.N. (2001) *Refugees and their Right to Communication: Perspective from South East Asia*, World Association for Christian Communication, London.
UNHCR (1951) Convention relating to the status of refugees, UNHCR, Geneva.

Notes

1   Between November 1989 and November 2001, 259 boats landed in Australia without authorisation, carrying a total of 13,489 people. Seventy per cent of those people arrived after July 1999 as smugglers began organising bigger boats carrying more passengers, representing a quantitative and qualitative shift in the nature of the problem. From mid 1999 onwards the average rate of arrival was around 335 people per month. However, immediately prior to the *Tampa* affair in August 2001, more than 1200 people arrived within the space of one month.
2   Australian Associated Press 13.9.2001.
3   For discussion of this issue see Henderson, Gerard 'Unleashing a "sleeper" issue: ethnic suspicion', the *Age*, 18.9.01.
4   See Atkins, Dennis 'PM links terror to asylum seekers' *Herald Sun* (Melbourne) 7.11.2001. For a defence of Howard's statement see Blair Tim, 'Beware of terrorists in refugee clothing', the *Australian* 8.11.01.
5   'Boat children overboard', the *Australian* 8.10.2001.
6   'Boat people "threw children overboard"', the *Age* 8.10.2001.
7   Reported by ABC online (www.abc.net.au) 9.8.02.
8   Personal interview with Peter Mares.
9   For a detailed critique of Australia's policies see Mares, Peter, *Borderline: Australia's treatment of refugees and asylum seekers*, UNSW Press, Sydney 2001.
10   'No human face for boat people', the *Age* 18.4.02.
11   See Smith and Harvey, 'Operation Safe Haven' in this volume.
12   Personal interview with the author Melbourne 5.7.2001.
13   Elizabeth Ferris—personal interview with the author Melbourne July 5, 2001.

Index